Respiratory Physiotherapy

For Elsevier:

Commissioning Editor: Rita Demetriou-Swanwick
Development Editor: Veronika Watkins
Project Manager: Kerrie-Anne Jarvis
Designer/Design Direction: George Ajayi
Illustrator: David Graham
Illustration Manager: Merlyn Harvey

Respiratory Physiotherapy: An On-Call Survival Guide

Second Edition

Edited by

Beverley Harden MSc, BSc (Hons), MCSP
Therapy Services Manager, Royal Hampshire County Hospital, Winchester

Dr Jane Cross EdD, MSc, Grad Dip Phys, MCSP
Senior Lecturer in Physiotherapy, University of East Anglia, Norwich

Mary-Ann Broad MSc (Critical care), BSc (Physiotherapy), MCSP
Clinical Specialist Physiotherapist, University Hospital of Wales, Cardiff

Matthew Quint MCSP, Grad Dip Phys, MPhil
Clinical Specialist Physiotherapist, Portsmouth City Teaching Primary Care Trust, Portsmouth

Paul Ritson MCSP
Clinical Specialist Physiotherapist, Paediatric Critical Care, Royal Liverpool Children's NHS Trust (Alder Hey), Liverpool

Sandy Thomas MEd, MCSP
Senior Lecturer, University of the West of England, Bristol

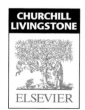

CHURCHILL
LIVINGSTONE

ELSEVIER

Edinburgh London New York Oxford Philadelphia St Louis Sydney Toronto 2009

CHURCHILL
LIVINGSTONE
ELSEVIER

© 2009, Elsevier Limited. All rights reserved.

No part of this publication may be reproduced or transmitted in any form or by any means, electronic or mechanical, including photocopying, recording, or any information storage and retrieval system, without permission in writing from the publisher. Permissions may be sought directly from Elsevier's Rights Department: phone: (+1) 215 239 3804 (US) or (+44) 1865 843830 (UK); fax: (+44) 1865 853333; e-mail: healthpermissions@elsevier.com. You may also complete your request on-line via the Elsevier website at http://www.elsevier.com/permissions.

First published 2004
Second edition 2009

ISBN: 978 0 7020 3003 1

British Library Cataloguing in Publication Data
A catalogue record for this book is available from the British Library

Library of Congress Cataloging in Publication Data
A catalog record for this book is available from the Library of Congress

Notice

Knowledge and best practice in this field are constantly changing. As new research and experience broaden our knowledge, changes in practice, treatment and drug therapy may become necessary or appropriate. Readers are advised to check the most current information provided (i) on procedures featured or (ii) by the manufacturer of each product to be administered, to verify the recommended dose or formula, the method and duration of administration, and contraindications. It is the responsibility of the practitioner, relying on their own experience and knowledge of the patient, to make diagnoses, to determine dosages and the best treatment for each individual patient, and to take all appropriate safety precautions. To the fullest extent of the law, neither the Publisher nor the Editors assumes any liability for any injury and/or damage to persons or property arising out or related to any use of the material contained in this book.

The Publisher

Printed in China

CONTENTS

Contributors viii

Foreword x

Acknowledgements xi

CHAPTER **1** **Learning for and from being on call** 1
Jane Cross

CHAPTER **2** **Practical on call preparation** 7
Mary-Ann Broad, Carole Jones

CHAPTER **3** **Respiratory assessment** 17
Matthew Quint, Sandy Thomas

CHAPTER **4** **Paediatric specifics** 37
Fiona Roberts

CHAPTER **5** **Chest X-ray interpretation** 51
Stephen Harden

CHAPTER **6** **The management of sputum retention** 71
Ruth Wakeman

CHAPTER **7** **The management of volume loss** 85
Bernadette Henderson, Nell Clotworthy

CHAPTER **8** **The management of increased work of breathing** 101
Alison Aldridge

CHAPTER **9** **Management of respiratory failure** 111
Sarah Keilty

CHAPTER **10**   **Calls to adult intensive care**   123
Rachel Devlin

CHAPTER **11**   **Calls to paediatric IUC (PICU)**   137
Elaine Dhouieb

CHAPTER **12**   **Calls to the medical unit**   145
Elizabeth Thomas

CHAPTER **13**   **Calls to the surgical ward**   159
Valerie Ball, Mary-Ann Broad

CHAPTER **14**   **Calls to the neurological/neurosurgical unit**   177
Lorraine Clapham

CHAPTER **15**   **Calls to the cardiothoracic unit**   189
Angela Kell

CHAPTER **16**   **Calls to the oncology unit**   205
Irelna Kruger, Katharine Malhotra

CHAPTER **17**   **Calls to the paediatric unit**   215
Paul Ritson

CHAPTER **18**   **Calls to the neonatal unit**   227
Alison Carter

CHAPTER **19**   **Respiratory physiotherapy treatments**   237
Alison Draper, Paul Ritson

CHAPTER **20**   **Case studies**   273
    1: Adult intensive care (*Rachel Devlin, Zoe Van Willigan*)
    2: Paediatric intensive care (*Elaine Dhouieb*)
    3: Medical unit (*Elizabeth Thomas*)
    4: Surgical unit (*Valerie Ball*)
    5: Neurological unit (*Lorraine Clapham*)
    6: Cardiothoracic unit (*Angela Kell*)
    7: Thoracic unit (*Angela Kell*)
    8: Haematology patient (*Irelna Kruger, Katharine Malhotra*)
    9: Oncology patient (*Irelna Kruger, Katharine Malhotra*)
    10: Paediatric ward (*Paul Ritson*)

APPENDIX **1** **Abbreviations** 293

APPENDIX **2** **Normal values** 297

APPENDIX **3** **Surgical incisions** 301

APPENDIX **4** **Common drugs used in critical care areas** 303
Angela Kell

Index 307

Alison Aldridge MCSP
Principal Respiratory Physiotherapist, Hampshire Primary Care Trust, Lymington

Valerie Ball MSc, MCSP
Lecturer, School of Health and Rehabilitation, Keele University, Keele

Mary-Ann Broad MSc (Critical care), BSc (Physiotherapy), MCSP
Clinical Specialist Physiotherapist, University Hospital of Wales, Cardiff

Alison Carter MCSP
Clinical Lead Acute Inpatient Paediatrics, Evelina Children's Hospital, Guy's and St Thomas' NHS Foundation Trust, London

Lorraine Clapham BSc (Hons), MCSP
Principal Clinical Lead Physiotherapist, Wessex Neurological Unit, Southampton

Nell Clotworthy MCSP, MSc
Clinical Specialist Respiratory Physiotherapist, South Devon Healthcare NHS Foundation Trust, Torbay Hospital, Torquay

Dr Jane Cross EdD, MSc, Grad Dip Phys, MCSP
Senior Lecturer in Physiotherapy, Univestity of East Anglia, Norwich

Rachel Devlin Grad Dip Phys, MCSP
Clinical Specialist Physiotherapist, General Intensive Care, Southampton University Hospitals NHS Trust, Southampton

Elaine Dhouieb MCSP, MSc
Respiratory Clinical Specialist, Physiotherapy Department, Royal Hospital for Sick Children, Edinburgh

Alison Draper MSc, MCSP, Cert HE
Lecturer, Division of Physiotherapy, School of Health Sciences, The University of Liverpool, Liverpool

Dr Stephen Harden MA, MB, BS, FRCS, FRCR
Consultant Cardiothoracic Radiologist, Wessex Cardiothoracic Centre, Southampton

Bernadette Henderson MSc, MCSP
Advanced Clinical Practitioner, Cardiorespiratory Physiotherapy, Barnet and Chase Farm NHS Trust, Barnet Hospital, Barnet

Carole Jones Grad Dip Phys, MCSP
Superintendent Physiotherapist, University Hospital of Wales, Cardiff

Sarah EJ Keilty MSc, MCSP
Consultant Physiotherapist, Respiratory & Critical Care, Guy's and St Thomas' NHS Foundation Trust, London

Angela Kell BSc (Hons), MCSP
Superintendent Physiotherapist, United Bristol Healthcare Trust, Physiotherapy Department, Bristol Royal Infirmary, Bristol

Irelna Kruger BSc, MCSP
Band 7 Physiotherapist, Royal Marsden NHS Foundation Trust, London

Katharine Malhotra BSc (Hons), MCSP
Superintendent Physiotherapist, Royal Marsden NHS Foundation Trust, London

Matthew Quint MCSP, Grad Dip Phys, MPhil
Clinical Specialist Physiotherapist, Portsmouth City Teaching Primary Care Trust, Portsmouth

Paul Ritson MCSP
Clinical Specialist Physiotherapist, Paediatric Critical Care, Royal Liverpool Children's NHS Trust (Alder Hey), Liverpool

Fiona Roberts MSc, BSc, MCSP
Lecturer in Physiotherapy, Faculty of Health and Social Care, School of Health Sciences, The Robert Gordon University, Aberdeen

Elizabeth Thomas MSc, Grad Dip Phys, MCSP
Medical Respiratory Lead Physiotherapist, Bradford Royal Infirmary, Bradford

Sandy Thomas MEd, MCSP
Senior Lecturer, University of the West of England, Bristol

Zoe Van Willigan BSc, MCSP
Band 7 Physiotherapist, General Intensive Care, Southampton University Hospitals NHS Trust, Southampton

Ruth Wakeman BSc (Physiotherapy), MCSP
Clinical Specialist Physiotherapist, Royal Brompton & Harefield NHS Trust, London

It is a privilege to have been invited to write the Foreword for the 2nd edition of the 'On-Call Survival Guide' for physiotherapists. The text has been edited by a team with extensive experience in respiratory physiotherapy, in the treatment of adults and children. Each chapter has been written by experienced clinicians with the knowledge to interpret and combine current evidence from the literature with clinical expertise, to optimise the physiotherapy assessment and management of the patient who is acutely ill.

The wealth of material encapsulated in this comprehensive text will help to alleviate the concerns of new physiotherapy graduates facing their first on-calls and of physiotherapists returning to the profession, both in preparing for the event and as guidance during the event. For those with more experience there is always something to be learned from our colleagues who may have more experience in managing certain problems or may have a different way of looking at a problem. This publication will help to establish and maintain physiotherapy as an essential component of healthcare.

Jennifer A Pryor PhD FNZSP MCSP

The Editors would like to thank everyone who has been involved in and has supported the creation of the second edition of this book and all those who supported the development of the first edition all those years ago. In particular, they acknowledge the contribution of the many physiotherapists who reviewed aspects of the manuscript:

Tom Bailey
Susanna Barr
Jennifer Bayliss
Louise Bowden
Helen Brewer
Em Butcher
Louisa Caile
Kate Cobley
Vanessa Compton
Lucy Coughlan
Judith Edwards
Rachel Ellis
Penny Galey
Helen Goldsmith
Sarah Goulding
Nick Harris
Nicola Henderson
Rachel Higgins
Jo Hobbs
Matthew Jones
Pip Kerr

Anne Konsta
Emma Larner
Emma Law
Christina Linton
Julia Lodge
Peter Lysakovia
Faye Mason
Daniel Meyrick
Jacqueline Mullan
Charlotte Murch
Corinne Robinson
Vikki Sanders
Claire Shaw
Christopher Smith
Zoe Stone
Jenny Tomkinson
Ann Touboulic
Eliza Wheeler
Lesley Wilbourn
Michael Wong

CHAPTER 1

Learning for and from being on call

Jane Cross

Many physiotherapists who work on call might feel uncertain whether they possess the skills and attributes required for this high-speed, complex environment. This service, like any other in the health service today, is subject to quality measures and standards. Clinical governance, as outlined in *The New NHS: Modern, Dependable* (DoH 1997), makes it clear that quality exists not only as a responsibility of the organization but also for each individual.

The intention of the following chapters is to provide the reader with insight into some of the ways in which you can assess your own learning needs, prepare for being on call and learn from each on call episode. Within the first chapter a number of tools that can help you in this process will be referred to. The description of these is necessarily brief and will not deal in detail with any of the particular tools suggested. Reference will be made to other work which develops these ideas further and could be used as a reading list. The second of the chapters lays out the practical preparation necessary prior to being on call.

Start by referring to your professional body to obtain the latest information on standards for on call working and the tools available to assist you in your continuing professional development. The Chartered Society of Physiotherapy has published *Emergency respiratory, on call working: guidance for physiotherapists*, Information paper no. PA53, London (2002). This document links the Core Standards of Physiotherapy to elements relevant to working in an on call setting; it is available to members at http://www.csp.org.uk/uploads/documents/csp_physioprac_pa531.pdf. The Association of Chartered Physiotherapists in Respiratory Care (ACPRC) On Call Project Team has produced an assessment tool (Thomas et al. 2006) which uses the elements of PA53 and has been designed to more specifically identify areas for development. It is available at http://www.acprc.org.uk/dmdocuments/competence_questionnaire.pdf and can be printed for use in your portfolio.

These sources will guide you through the process.

HOW CAN WE PREPARE FOR AN ON CALL EVENT?

Reflect:

● What do you know already?

● What do you need to know?

Spend a moment thinking about what you already know and what you need to know. Reflection is about learning from experience (Spalding 1998) and as such is a valuable tool for the practitioner from the perspective of their own professional development.

Reflection

Further reading which is presented as a personal experience of using reflection to demonstrate professional development can be found in Spalding (1998).

● Complete a SWOT analysis.

SWOT analysis

Tools such as a SWOT analysis (strengths, weaknesses, opportunities and threats) can be useful in this process. For further information and an illustration of the use of this tool see Atkinson (1998). Alternatively you can use the on call competency checklist.

The process of producing a SWOT analysis/using the on call competency checklist can be undertaken as a piece of individual reflection. However, these could also be facilitated by a peer. Ask someone to help you. A colleague could help you recognize some of the strengths, weaknesses, etc. that you have in relation to working on call.

Once you are clear upon what your needs are and recognize some of your strengths, it may be useful to set up a learning contract with yourself and/or your manager or senior member of staff, as appropriate. Alternatively add these needs to your existing personal development plan (PDP).

Learning contracts

This contract should identify the means by which an individual can achieve their identified learning needs. These means could include work experience opportunities, teaching sessions that they would like to attend, internally organized training programmes as well as external courses and perhaps more formal routes of academic learning. This list is by no means exhaustive. Individuals and their managers should be as innovative as possible when trying to identify the means of meeting these learning needs. The more formalized external routes of leaning should only be contemplated when internal resources cannot meet these needs. Included within the contract should be review dates and evaluative measures. For more information regarding learning contracts see Walker (1999).

● Arrange for an induction.

Talk to those who work in the areas you are likely to be called into. Arrange to spend some time with them. You may need a guided tour of where equipment is kept, or a quick talk through some of the processes operated on individual wards. Spend some time on the intensive care unit (ICU) and high dependency unit (HDU) so that you can see the equipment in use and meet some of the staff who work there.

Try to meet some of these needs before your first on call event but recognize some of these will take longer to fulfil than others!

HOW CAN WE LEARN FROM THE ON CALL EVENT?

● Recording your thoughts following your on call, either as a critical incident or as part of your reflective diary, will form a useful record of your thoughts and feelings at this time. This record will help you recognize your learning needs for the future but also, and possibly more importantly, it will help you recognize the progress you are making in your efforts to enhance your competence.

● Follow your on call event up with a 'debrief' either as a paper exercise for yourself or with a colleague or the senior member of staff with responsibility for on call. Use your skills of reflection to learn from this recent experience.

Ask

● How did it go?
● What went well?
● What could have gone better?
● Why do you think that particular aspect went well/not so well?
● How could you improve upon that aspect?
● What do you need to do in order to improve that aspect?
● How can that be facilitated?
● Do you need any resources in order to achieve this?

Answering these questions may help you to reflect upon your experience and identify what you have learned and what further learning you need to undertake to achieve the enhanced competence that you seek.

If you choose to 'debrief' with another person certain criteria need to be met to ensure that this is a learning event. The person with whom you undertake this debriefing/reflection must be able to support you in a non-threatening way. Their role is to facilitate you in your thinking about your clinical reasoning and your resulting actions. They need to help you identify what went well and what could have been improved. By doing this you can then identify ongoing learning needs and identify ways in which these can be achieved.

● Use your learning diary to facilitate this period of reflection with another therapist.
● Use your learning diary to facilitate your own individual and internalized reflective activity.

Learning diary/learning log

The use of a learning diary, in which a clinician records on call situations, their actions, the clinical reasoning which led to these actions and their feelings about the situation, could be used as a record from which an individual could demonstrate their competency. It could actually be referred to as written-down reflection. Furthermore, it can be used as a useful learning tool. For example, if excerpts from this were used during a debriefing (reflection), following an on call episode, this process could be turned into a learning event.

Critical incident report (this is within the context of learning, not risk management!)

Incidents such as these occur throughout our working lives. They do not have to be awful moments; they can be really positive moments when we know we have done something really well. Alternatively they could be 'ah ha' moments, such as when the penny drops when battling to understand a difficult concept or skill that we have been grappling with for a while. Recording these moments can help us identify how and what we have learned from a given situation or moment. Recording these can help us later, as a record of what it was we felt we had achieved. They can also facilitate our 'reflection on action' (Schon 1991), which is the term coined for thinking about an incident some time after it has occurred to identify what went well/wrong so that we can learn more from it and thus move on further in our learning process.

● Include a critical incident analysis in your learning diary.

HOW CAN WE DEMONSTRATE WHAT WE HAVE LEARNED?

Use the tools we have identified to create a section in your portfolio which can be used to demonstrate the competencies you have demonstrated.

Portfolio

This is a collection of material that we can present to demonstrate to others that we have achieved the learning that we set out to do. This planned learning can be evidenced by including, in a portfolio, SWOT analyses and learning contracts. Evidence that this learning has been achieved could include extracts from learning diaries/logs, critical incident reports, anonymous case study reports, extracts from courses, training sessions attended, etc. It is important, however, with this type of collection of evidence that the individual remembers that they will be bringing this into the public arena. Particular attention should thus be paid to maintaining the confidentiality both of others – professional and patient – and of ourselves. Further reading can be found in Stewart (1998).

● Participate in some case studies where you can use real or imaginary cases to demonstrate your clinical reasoning. You could also use these in preparation for on call to practise your clinical reasoning.

Case studies

Sound clinical reasoning is one such skill that is essential for safe practice across the spectrum of physiotherapy work. This is one of the hardest areas to assess regarding the competency issue. Using case studies in on call/respiratory in-service education is one way in which clinicians can assess competency in this area. Real or imaginary case studies can be used to examine the clinical reasoning process in a variety of settings and covering a variety of topics. Both the educator and the learner can take responsibility for producing these and they can be used as a record for an individual's portfolio. For further reading about using clinical reasoning as a tool for demonstrating continuing professional development see Stephenson (1998).

● Undertake peer review with a colleague. You could choose to work on a case together or use incidents from your learning diary or a critical incident.
● Link closely with your mentor to develop your learning.

Peer review

This is another method by which the clinician can assess their own and others' competency. This tool could be used both in the here-and-now by treating a real patient and when going through the reasoning with a colleague who is present both during the treatment and afterwards. Incidents from your learning log or critical incident reports could also be the stimulus for discussion. This can follow on from the use of case studies as outlined earlier.

Ground rules need to be established and agreed before these sessions take place and these should include how an individual would like to receive feedback, the confidentiality that is to be expected on the part of both the reviewed and the reviewer, and what type of record of the session is to be kept.

Following the ideas in this chapter can help you prepare well for your first on call event, plan your learning and record your achievements. This should help you as adult learners to take responsibility for your own learning and empower you to ask for the support that you need to achieve both confidence and competence in an on call situation.

References

Atkinson K (1998) SWOT analysis: a tool for continuing professional development. BJTR 5(8):433–435.

Department of Health (1997) White Paper. The New NHS: Modern, Dependable. London: HMSO.

Schon D (1991) The reflective practitioner: how professionals think in action, 2nd edn. San Francisco, CA: Jossey Bass.

Spalding N (1998) Reflection in professional development: a personal experience. BJTR 5(7):379–382.

Stephenson R (1998) Can clinical reasoning be an effective tool in CPD? BJTR 5(6):325–329.

Stewart S (1998) The place of portfolios in continuing professional development. BJTR 5(5):266–269.

Thomas S, Broad MA, Cross J, Harden B, Quint M, Ritson P (2006) Acute Respiratory/On Call Physiotherapy – Self-evaluation of competence questionnaire. Available online: www.acprc.org.uk/dmdocuments/competence_questionnaire.pdf

Walker E (1999) Learning contracts in practice: their role in CPD. BJTR 6(2):91–94.

CHAPTER 2

Practical on call preparation

Mary-Ann Broad and Carole Jones

This chapter suggests how you can prepare and learn from your experiences to guide your continuing professional development (CPD). Senior staff are able to facilitate your learning needs but it is *your* personal responsibility to ensure you are competent. There are some areas you can read up on and prepare in advance; others will need the support of your senior colleagues. Each department is different and you will be able to get information pertinent to your hospital from your manager.

Remember – BE PREPARED!

THINGS TO CONSIDER PRIOR TO BEING ON CALL:
- On call policy/procedures
- Infection control
- Identification of your learning needs
- Clinical experience
- Training/induction
- Shadow duties.

On call policy/procedures
Request a copy of the departmental policy. Read this carefully; it will include valuable information on the operational aspects of the service, such as:
- *On call period*, e.g. 5 pm–9 am. You must be free to respond to a call at any time within that period.
- *Referral criteria*. There should be clear guidelines for staff regarding the clinical needs of patients who should be referred.
- *Response time*. You should be able to respond within a given time. If not, you will need to stay in hospital accommodation. Discuss this with your manager to help you access an on call room if appropriate.
- *Health and safety issues*, e.g. parking and accessing the department at night, working alone, the availability of personal alarms, taxis, infection control, etc.

● There are likely to be other contractual issues, e.g. payment, time in lieu arrangements and organization of the rota local to your hospital.

Infection control

Before you are on call, read your organization's infection control policy. Remember that policies vary between organizations and over time.

Sick patients will have a reduced capacity to overcome further infection and may have numerous points (drips/drains/catheters) for infection to be introduced. Exercise universal precautions for all patients and check for instructions if you are called to a patient being nursed in isolation.

Remember your own protection in terms of risk assessment; drips, drains and attachments produce an increased risk of contact with body fluids and exposure to bloodborne pathogens. More notably, physiotherapy techniques can increase the quantity of respiratory pathogens exhaled into room air. Ensure you know what precautions are expected in addition to universal precautions and where you can access the protective equipment required. Be aware of local policy for management of a needlestick injury or splash incident to the eyes/mouth.

> **Remember**
> If you are unsure which precautions to use, ask before commencing an assessment.
>
> Be aware of your own vaccination record and how additional health factors (e.g. your own early pregnancy) might influence your risk assessment.

Identification of your learning needs

There should be an opportunity formally to assess your knowledge and skills with a senior clinician. This will ensure that you have a basic level of competence prior to commencing on call and will facilitate identification of learning needs and subsequent development plans. You are expected to have learning needs – qualification as a physiotherapist does not mean you are fully competent or you feel confident to work on call!

It is useful to have done some preparation to identify your own learning needs; refer to Chapter 1.

Clinical experience

Your hospital should provide you with an on call induction, which will offer opportunities to experience different clinical specialities. It is often not possible to have a rotation which includes critical care prior to joining the on call rota, therefore maximize your learning opportunities during your induction. Remember many skills are transferable.

Familiarize yourself with the following:

- Geography of the hospital and wards
- Treatment guidelines/protocols for your hospital
- Contraindications/precautions to treatment
- Clinical workload – you can do this by working alongside a mentor:
  - Observe and discuss assessment
  - Discuss clinical reasoning/problem solving
  - Observe the application of treatment modalities and their evaluation/ modification if necessary
- Location and assembly of equipment:
  - e.g. IPPB, suction catheters, humidification, and how to access it at night
  - Practise under supervision as systems will vary from Trust to Trust
- How to access patient information.

On call training/induction

Alongside your individualized learning in the clinical environment each department should have ongoing learning opportunities involving workshops and lectures designed to update staff on key respiratory topics. It is your responsibility to revise your basic anatomy and physiology.

Shadow duties

Some hospitals offer the opportunity to 'shadow' a senior colleague on call, prior to being on call independently. Use this opportunity to:

- Observe the on call procedure, e.g. contacting the switchboard, travelling, parking, attending the call and discussing the case, recording attendance/ documentation, claiming payment, etc.
- As your confidence builds, take the lead with the support and guidance of your mentor. Discuss your clinical reasoning, proposed treatment plan or any problems you have encountered. You may now feel confident with their support on the phone.

ON CALL ROTA

Once you are on the on call rota there are elements you can prepare for including:

- On call logistics
- Management of the telephone call
- Understanding appropriate and inappropriate calls.

On call logistics

On the day of your on call:

- Were there any calls during the previous night? If so, are further call outs to this patient required? Has the patient improved with treatment through the course of the day? If possible review/treat the patient with the appropriate clinician.
- Identify patients who may require on call, liaise with senior colleagues and review them if possible.
- Prioritize and discuss your own caseload with your senior ensuring cover for the next day; this will be determined by your local European Working Time Directive agreement.
- Before leaving work, contact the hospital switchboard to advise them of your points of contact (pager and/or telephone). It is good practice to give two points of contact.
- Remember to take with you:
  - A (confidential) list of contact numbers for the senior clinicians
  - A copy of the on call referral criteria
  - A list of questions to ask if called (to allow you to remain focused despite any underlying panic!). See management of the telephone call below
  - Your uniform, stethoscope, pager or phone.

Management of the telephone call

Think ahead, a proforma can be used to guide your questions over the telephone (Fig. 2.1). Many hospitals may also provide a list of on call questions. These will provide a brief outline of the patient's condition.

Advice to consider whilst on the telephone

It may be appropriate to give advice over the phone prior to you arriving on the ward. This may include:

- Positioning – for drainage, V/Q matching or to reduce work of breathing
- Pain control – is this adequate? Do they need more analgesia prior to physio?
- Bronchodilators – are they prescribed and could the patient have a dose?
- Could nebulized saline be considered?
- O_2 therapy – is this being delivered appropriately? Should the patient be on a humidified circuit? If saturations are low can this be increased. (Remember this should be agreed with the doctor.)

Staff may also call seeking advice where attendance by the on call physiotherapist is not appropriate. You should still gain an accurate history of the patient and give

Patient's name:	
Location:	
Referred by:	
Admitted with:	
What has happened/current status:	
Previous history of note:	
CNS Level of consciousness/GCS, ?sedated	
CVS Stable? Parameters in normal range?	
Renal Adequate urine output? Fluid balance?	
RS Ventilation, RR, SpO_2, FiO_2 requirements, ABGs, CXR	
Additional questions: • Patient's position • ?Dr's review • Suction • Contraindications/cautions	
Previous physio treatment and effect?	
Current assessment findings	
Primary problem	
Appropriate referral? Why?	
Treatment/advice details	

Figure 2.1 On call prompt sheet.

advice as you feel appropriate. Check with your local policy on documentation of these calls.

Appropriate and inappropriate calls

In some hospitals a senior medical doctor must call out the on call physiotherapist. In others, all calls to the critical care unit must be attended – check the local policy for your hospital.

Many conditions benefit from physiotherapy, but for some it is unlikely to help. In many cases the referrer is asking for a second opinion/assessment; this is an appropriate part of patient care. Table 2.1 summarizes some examples of appropriate and inappropriate calls in the on call setting. These lists are not exhaustive and every call must be assessed on its own merits.

The telephone conversation should give you a clearer clinical picture. If you feel the request is inappropriate, explain your reasons and discuss them with the person calling. If the situation is unclear despite your best efforts or the referrer does not agree that physiotherapy is not indicated, you should attend to assess the patient in order to determine the exact clinical picture and need for treatment. Remember, this is an emergency service for patients who would significantly deteriorate without treatment.

Table 2.1 Examples of appropriate and inappropriate calls

Conditions where physiotherapy can help	Conditions where physiotherapy is unlikely to help
<ul><li>Recent aspiration</li><li>Recent atelectasis/collapse</li><li>Retained secretions causing respiratory distress, e.g. pneumonia, bronchiectasis, CF, COPD with infection or secretions following recent extubation</li><li>Poor cough associated with infection and unable to clear</li><li>Non-encapsulated lung abscess that will respond to postural drainage</li><li>Patients that have benefited from intensive respiratory treatment throughout the day</li></ul>	<ul><li>Pulmonary oedema – unless infected</li><li>Pulmonary embolus</li><li>Pulmonary fibrosis</li><li>ARDS with minimal secretions</li><li>Non-acute, non-productive COPD</li><li>Non-productive consolidated infection, e.g. TB, pneumonia</li><li>Empyema, pleural effusion, pneumothorax – perhaps beneficial if chest drain inserted</li><li>Encapsulated lung abscess</li><li>Acute bronchospasm, e.g. asthma unless associated with sputum retention</li><li>Patients coughing and expectorating unaided</li></ul>

THINGS TO CONSIDER WHEN YOU ARE CALLED IN TO A PATIENT

First things first – look at the patient! (refer to assessment chapters). The following elements must be considered – and prior preparation is suggested.

- Communication
- Consent
- Dealing with children
- Documentation and feedback.

Communication

General communication with the medical/nursing staff

You may need to act quickly to prevent further deterioration of an unwell patient. Other members of the team can give you valuable information for your assessment:

- Speak to the nurse responsible for the patient to gain more detail on the patient's history and recent deterioration.
- Did any of the advice you gave improve the patient's condition or has the patient continued to deteriorate since they called you?
- Do you need the nurse to assist you with your assessment or treatment?
- Contact the doctor if required.
- Ascertain the patient's resuscitation status. If the patient is unstable there is a risk of respiratory or cardiac arrest during your treatment. Check in the nursing or medical notes. If you are unclear, discuss with nursing staff or doctor. Make sure that this is the most recent decision.

Communication with the patient/relatives

- Explain your role to the patient – this can reduce anxiety and distress.
- If relatives are present, ask the patient (if possible) whether or not they would like the relatives present during treatment.
- Relatives sometimes express concern about the proposed treatment, despite a full explanation. In this situation, seek the guidance of the doctor, who may need to clarify the situation with the relatives.

Should clinicians disagree?

Professional autonomy allows physiotherapists the freedom to decide not to treat patients in situations where it is assessed that treatment is inappropriate/contra-indicated, despite the doctor's request.

- Discuss your concerns with the doctor.
- Why does the doctor feel that treatment is indicated?
- Could further investigations, such as chest X-ray, be performed to give clarity to the situation?

If you are still unhappy, you may wish to phone a senior physiotherapist for support and guidance.

When to seek help
Remember that other members of the multidisciplinary team and your senior colleagues are there to support you. You must recognize your scope of practice. In certain situations you should seek their support:

● If the patient is deteriorating rapidly.
● Following assessment you consider the patient is too unstable to tolerate treatment and may require transfer to critical care for further medical management.
● Following assessment you are unable to identify the problem and are uncertain about appropriate management.
● You are unsure about specific modifications required for a planned treatment (e.g. the patient has recently undergone upper GI surgery and suction is indicated).
● You have identified the problem but feel that the required treatment is outside your scope of practice.

Consent

● There is a legal requirement where at all possible to obtain consent to treat. Consent may be written, verbal or non-verbal and should be documented in the patient's treatment record. Be aware of your own organization's policy on consent.
● We have a duty to provide appropriate information so that consent is informed (i.e. the patient must be aware of the implications of treatment and any possible side-effects).
● Mentally competent adult patients are entitled to refuse treatment, even when it would clearly benefit their health. The only exception is where the treatment is for a mental disorder and the patient is detained under the Mental Health Act 1983.

Remember
Do not attempt to resolve complex issues of consent on your own.

Patients without capacity
Some adult patients may lack sufficient mental capacity to make specific decisions at the time they need to be made. In these circumstances, these adults may not be able to provide valid informed consent or withhold consent to the proposed treatment.

The Mental Capacity Act 2005, covering Wales and England, provides the legal framework for acting and making decisions on behalf of individuals aged 16 and over who lack the mental capacity to make particular decisions for themselves. The Adults with Incapacity (Scotland) Act 2000 provides a similar framework for Scotland.

The Act has five statutory principles:
1. Assume that a person has capacity unless there is evidence otherwise.
2. Support a person, as far as practicable, to make their own decision.
3. Do not treat a person as lacking capacity because a decision is unwise.
4. All decisions must be in the best interests of a person who lacks capacity.
5. Consider less restrictive alternatives before making a decision.

To help determine if a person lacks capacity to make particular decisions, the Act sets out a two-stage test of capacity:

Stage 1: Does the person have an impairment of, or a disturbance in the functioning of, their mind or brain?

Stage 2: Does the impairment or disturbance mean that the person is unable to make a specific decision when they need to?

A person is unable to make a decision if they cannot:
1. Understand information about the decision to be made
2. Retain that information
3. Use or weigh that information as part of the decision-making process
4. Communicate their decision (verbal, non-verbal or other).

The Act also provides guidance for working out the best interests of a person who lacks capacity to make a particular decision, to allow decisions about medical treatment or social care to be made on their behalf in the absence of valid informed consent. The Act allows health and social care staff to carry out certain tasks in connection with care and treatment on behalf of someone believed to lack capacity to give, or withhold, permission for the action. The Act provides protection from liability for these actions provided the person who is going to take the action has a reasonable belief that the individual lacks capacity and reasonable grounds for believing that the action is in the best interests of the person who lacks capacity.

An advance decision made under the Mental Capacity Act enables someone aged 18 and over, while still mentally capable, to refuse medical treatment for a time in the future when they may lack the capacity to consent to or refuse that treatment. Healthcare professionals will be protected from liability if they stop or withhold treatment because they reasonably believe that an advance decision to refuse treatment exists and that it is valid and applicable.

2

A power of attorney is a legal document that allows one person to give another person authority to make a decision on their behalf. It is possible for a person aged 18 and over with mental capacity (the donor) to make a Lasting Power of Attorney (LPA) that can be used to appoint an attorney (the donee) to make decisions about personal welfare, which can include healthcare and medical treatment decisions. A personal welfare LPA can be used only at a time when the donor lacks capacity to make a specific welfare decision.

These situations should be clearly documented in the patient's treatment records and any queries discussed with the medical team.

Information on the Mental Capacity Act and consent issues within the UK is available from http://www.dh.gov.uk/en/Policyandguidance/Healthandsocialcaretopics/Consent/index.htm.

Dealing with children

The paediatric chapters will provide you with invaluable information on consent in children and for managing this patient group.

Documentation and feedback

Document your assessment/treatment/outcome and when the patient will next be reviewed in the medical notes. This should include the date and time of the call and who called you in. When signing the notes include your name in block capitals, your job title and a contact number (e.g. bleep number). Check with local policy for documentation standards.

It is important to give feedback to the patient, relatives and other professionals:

● Discuss the outcome of your assessment and/or treatment with the nursing staff. Let them know when the patient will be reviewed and under what circumstances they should call you again.
● Advise how nursing staff can maintain improvement (e.g. positioning, nebulized saline, suction).
● Discuss with the patient or relatives when you will next review.
● It is courteous to contact the normal ward physiotherapist to hand over the patient and when they need review the next day.

Acknowledgement

Specific thanks to Dorian Davies BA, PGCE, DipSW, Mental Capacity Act Implementation Manager Cardiff and Vale NHS Trust for his assistance on the consent and capacity section.

CHAPTER 3

Respiratory assessment

Matthew Quint and Sandy Thomas

The primary goal is to establish the clinical situation, the indications for and contra-indications to treatment. This starts from the moment the referral is received. Not all information is required for all patients so tailor your assessment to the patient.

In any clinical situation a 'quick check' from the end of the bed can be crucial in establishing the stability of the patient and direct you as to how quickly you should act and how ill the patient is. Although you will want to focus on physiotherapy problems and treatment strategies, your first priority is to ensure patient safety; therefore, your first question should be: 'Is the patient in immediate danger?' Assess by reviewing:

Patient A

● It is 20.00 hrs and you are called to see an 84-year-old gentleman on a medical ward. He was admitted yesterday with a community-acquired pneumonia and was treated earlier in the day by the ward physiotherapist. The sister reports he has dropped his oxygen saturation and sounds bubbly. She has asked that you review this patient.

● He has a previous stroke and mild dementia. While he is for full and active treatment, he is not considered appropriate for resuscitation

● On arrival at the ward, the registrar is reviewing the notes, and the nursing staff are handing over to the night staff.

What should you do now?

● **A – Airway**, is it patent and protected? What are their oxygen saturations and are they on oxygen?
  ● If not: Call for help and establish an airway.

- **B – Breathing**, are they ventilating effectively?
  - If not: Call for help and support ventilation.
- **C – Circulation**, do they have an adequate cardiac output?
  - If not: Call for help and support output.

If the answer to any of these questions is 'no' something immediately needs to be done to stabilize the patient. Could *you* recognize these signs and would *you* know how to address them? If not, you require an update on basic life support. Refer also to respiratory and circulatory sections within this chapter. Therefore, for Patient A, start with ABC, then perform a full assessment.

Patient A had audible crackles at the mouth, was using his accessory muscles and was breathing very shallowly. It was clear that his airway was compromised and needed to be cleared immediately to ensure his safety before the assessment could proceed.

If you are unsure – do not be afraid to call for help.

Remember you do not have sole responsibility for the care of the patient. Other members of the team are there to support you, just as you are there to support them.

Once you have established that the patient is in no immediate danger, your next goal should be to find out whether the patient has (or is at risk of developing) one or more of the following four key problems:

- Sputum retention
- Loss of lung volume
- Increased work of breathing
- Respiratory failure.

Management of each of these problems is summarized in individual chapters and the decision-making process is shown in Fig. 3.1.

You should be systematic in your approach and include each physiological system: cardiovascular, renal, etc.

SUBJECTIVE HISTORY

Consider: What has changed? Why has it changed? How does this impact on the patient and/or the clinical intervention?

HISTORY OF PRESENT CONDITION

Reflect on whether the patient's current situation might be related to any of the four key physiotherapy problems. You can also determine the 'trend' of the problem/symptoms and whether the patient is deteriorating, stable or improving since the onset.

Focus on the key symptoms: wheeze, shortness of breath, cough, sputum and chest pain.

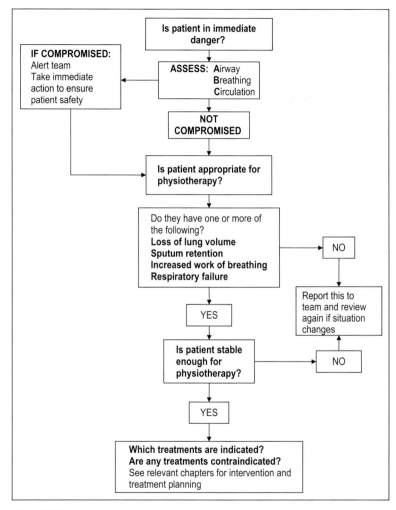

Figure 3.1 Decision-making process.

3

Wheeze

What may be the cause (swelling, bronchospasm or sputum)? What is most likely to be the case with your patient (are there any clues in the PMH)?

Shortness of breath

If shortness of breath at rest (or on minimal exercise) is not normal for the patient, this is cause for concern and could lead to fatigue if not addressed. What can you do to relieve the work of breathing?

Cough

A cough is a normal and important part of airway clearance, both reflex and under voluntary control. Is it effective? Productive or dry? Is the patient wasting energy on an unproductive cough and getting fatigued? Remember that a cough will only clear the central airways.

Sputum

How much, what colour, how viscous, is it difficult to clear? Does the patient normally have an airway clearance regimen and is it working?

Chest pain

Cardiac chest pain is likely to be crushing and central, radiating to the left arm and neck (if recent onset this should be highlighted to the team). For other sources of pain ensure there is adequate analgesia to allow treatment.

PAST MEDICAL HISTORY

You are trying to establish how serious the current episode is for this patient, and whether you can draw on past experience to find the most effective treatment. Think about:

● Underlying pathologies that may impact on the patient's care?
● Contraindications to treatment?
● Any allergies?
● Previous/similar episodes?
● What treatment has the patient had before?
● Has the patient required physiotherapy before and how did they respond?

DRUG HISTORY

This should also include oxygen prescription. Often patients will report they are fit and well, but on questioning report a long list of medications that highlight other pathologies (Table 3.1).

Table 3.1 Drug history

● Normal medications?	● Does this tell you about any further PMH?
● Current medications?	● Is there any other drug that could facilitate physiotherapy, e.g. nebulized normal saline?

SOCIAL HISTORY

What is the patient normally like? Is there a history of smoking? Remember that smoking is the major cause of chronic lung disease.

OBJECTIVE HISTORY

You now need to identify the current situation. Look for trends over time. Is the patient compromised, improving, unchanged or deteriorating? The two key components to this section of the assessment are:

● Observation – including charts
● Physical examination.

Remember it is all too easy to dive in but it is important to take a considered approach (Table 3.2).

Table 3.2 Considered approach to assessment

STOP	Take stock of the situation and what you have discovered so far
LOOK	Look at the patient carefully and the information available from the charts and monitors
LISTEN	Listen to what the patient tells you and to what you hear on auscultation
FEEL	Examine them systematically. Remember your hands may tell you far more than a stethoscope
THINK	Relate your findings to the patient's history. What potential problems have you identified and are they consistent with the history? Can you manage this patient or do you need help?

This approach should be used as you work through the various systems (Tables 3.3–3.7).

General observation provides an opportunity to take in the overall situation of the patient including the equipment surrounding them, the personnel and any relatives or carers (Table 3.3). While issues of consent and treatment should be directed to the patient, you may need to involve others in discussions.

Table 3.3 **General observations**

Comfort	Does the patient look comfortable, or unwell and distressed; do you need to deal with this first?
Size	Are they obese? What are the manual handling and respiratory implications of this? Alternatively if malnourished they may fatigue quickly
Position	What position do you find them in? This has a real impact on lung volumes and work of breathing (see Chapter 7)
Posture	Do they have a kyphosis or scoliosis? Chest wall deformity may be associated with loss of volume and respiratory failure (see Chapters 7 and 9)
Apparatus	What equipment, drains or lines are attached to the patient; are they switched on and are they working properly? **If you are unfamiliar with the equipment: Ask**

CARDIOVASCULAR SYSTEM

This will give you more information regarding the patient's stability and ability to tolerate physiotherapy. Remember, things may change quickly so keep monitoring for any deterioration.

- Look for trends
- What is their normal status?
- What physiological stress is the patient under?
- Is their circulation becoming compromised?

Table 3.4 **Cardiovascular observations**

Observations	Relevance
Heart rate ● Bradycardia HR <50/min Tachycardia HR >100/min	Consider predicted 'maximum' (220 − age): does the patient have enough reserve for physiotherapy?
Blood pressure ● Normal 95/60–140/90 mmHg	Increases with age. Significance of abnormal values depends on patient's normal. Note changes or trends
● Hypotension <95/60 (adults)	A patient whose pulse is higher than their systolic blood pressure at rest is significantly compromised This needs to be addressed quickly by members of the team Ideally avoid physiotherapy until pressure stable
● Hypertension >140/90 (adults)	Significance depends on patient's age and their usual values. A diastolic >95 mmHg warrants a degree of caution
● Inotropic drugs	The cardiovascular system may be less stable so take care with treatments (See Chapters 10, 15 and Appendix 4)

Table 3.4 *Continued*

Observations	Relevance
Central venous pressure (CVP)	Gives an indication of overall fluid filling and is measured invasively via a central line Low values – patient may be dehydrated or have poor venous return High values – may be due to positive pressure ventilation, fluid overload or heart failure
Capillary refill time (CRT)	Measured by pinching a finger at the level of the heart and holding for 5 seconds. Count how long it takes for blanching to clear. Normal ≤3 seconds. Longer suggests poor blood flow which could be related to inadequate circulation overall ***Remember***, *just feeling the peripheries will give you an idea of how well perfused the patient is – the colder the worse the circulation*
Oedema	Oedema to both legs might suggest heart failure. Generalized oedema may also affect the lungs and present as crackles which sound similar to sputum retention, but will not respond to physiotherapy treatment
Haematological values	If WCC increased, suggests an infection If platelets lowered, may increase risk of bleeding and contraindicate manual techniques. Note the clotting time/INR
Temperature	Look for hyper- or hypothermia – either could compromise patient's tolerance of intervention

ECG MONITORING

You are not responsible for diagnosis – ask for help if unsure. If something does not look right, do ask – you may be the first person to have seen a new problem. First check the 'stickies' or ECG dots and leads are still attached. Look to see if trace is regular, and if it's fast or slow. A serious dysrhythmia in one person may have no adverse effects in another, so look at the patient! Blood pressure is *the key* when deciding the importance of any dysrhythmia. Also consider general observations such as colour, temperature and conscious level. Any *trend* of the dysrhythmia is also important.

● Has it just occurred?
● Did it occur suddenly or gradually?

3

● Is it getting more frequent?
● How is your treatment affecting it?

Pay attention to dysrhythmias that have recently appeared, or are getting more frequent. Remember, manual chest treatments may affect the ECG tracing, so allow time for the tracing to settle before interpreting any abnormality.

NEUROLOGICAL SYSTEM

This is considered in more detail in Chapter 14.

There remains some debate as to the most effective and quick assessment of neurological status. Some units will opt for 'AVPU' and others will use GCS. You should abide by local guidelines.

Table 3.5 Neurological observations

Observations	Relevance
AVPU ● A quick and easy assessment of a patient's overall neurological status	**A** = patient is **A**lert **V** = responds to **V**oice **P** = only responds to **P**ain **U** = **U**nresponsive If patient's status is lower than 'Alert', is the team aware of this? If not, report immediately Take note if the neurological status deteriorates during your assessment/treatment and alert team Unresponsive patients need their airway protected – consider oral airway, or recovery position where appropriate
GCS ● Glasgow Coma Scale ● A more detailed assessment of neurological status scored between 3 and 15	It tests best response of: Eyes (scored 1–4) Verbal (scored 1–5) Motor (scored 1–6) Is most useful for those familiar with its scoring If there is a change in the total GCS score alert medical and nursing colleagues
Pupils	Look at size and reactivity. Pinpoint pupils may suggest too much morphine. Unequal pupils may indicate neurological changes
Neurological observations ● ICP and CPP	See Chapter 14 Report any change Use to monitor adverse effects of physiotherapy

Table 3.5 *Continued*

Observations	Relevance
Drugs: sedation	Is patient receiving any sedative drugs? What is the level of sedation (does your hospital score sedation levels)? Sedation may affect ability to participate in treatment or may be needed if patient is agitated Heavily sedated patients may not be able to cooperate with active treatments (e.g. ACBT)
Drugs: paralysing	Is the patient receiving any paralysing agents? Paralysed patients cannot breathe for themselves Take extra care when removing from ventilator to bag and when moving patient (e.g. joint protection, reassurance)
Tone	Changes in tone or patterning give some idea of severity of neurological damage and implications for moving the patient. How do they handle?
Blood glucose ● Normal level 4–6 mmol/L	Low values impair patient's neurological status. May need to be addressed immediately
Pain	Are they in pain? Is a scoring system being used? What analgesia is being used? What dose? What route? Is it adequate? Ask for pain control to be increased for physiotherapy if necessary

RENAL SYSTEM

Patients with renal failure can require a variety of forms of support. This frequently involves the insertion of large-bore cannulae (e.g. Vas-Cath). Care must be taken while handling patients that these are not occluded or dislodged.

Table 3.6 Renal observations

Observations	Relevance
Urine output ● Normal output 0.5–1.0 ml per kg body weight per hour	Just because there is no urine output, this does not necessarily mean the patient is in renal failure. Is there a catheter in situ, is it blocked, is it in the right place? Poor output may be related to shock and risk of cardiovascular insufficiency – need to discuss with team
Fluid balance chart ● Look at cumulative balance, i.e. input vs. output (check totals include all sources of fluid loss)	*Remember* – *Change in urine output is a sensitive marker of patient improvement or deterioration* Check for low albumin levels which may be associated with circulatory compromise despite an apparently normal fluid balance Overhydration (risk of pulmonary oedema and crackles that are not due to sputum) Underhydration (risk of dehydration and viscous sputum)

MUSCULOSKELETAL

Key questions to ask:

● Is there a history of trauma past or present? Will this impact on your planned treatment?

● Is there a potential spinal fracture or has the spine been 'cleared'? If unsure treat as unstable – see Chapter 14.

● Injuries can be missed initially so do not be surprised if you discover additional injuries (e.g. ligamentous disruption) and ensure they are reported.

● Identify any fractures, soft tissue injuries and how they are being managed. External fixators and traction may limit how you can position the patient.

RESPIRATORY

These observations should guide you towards any key physiotherapy problems (Table 3.7).

Airway should always be assessed first – Is it patent and protected? If there is an airway, what type is there – endotracheal tube, tracheostomy, nasal or oral airway?

Table 3.7 Respiratory observations

Observations	Relevance
Mode of ventilation	Spontaneous, non-invasive or invasive? (NIV see Chapter 9, Invasive ventilation see Chapter 10)
Respiratory rate ● Adult normal 12–16	Compare documented rate to rate that *you* measure. Expect increases when demand increases
● Increased RR	Check $PaCO_2$ – if low the patient could be hyperventilating Due to stress? Anxiety? Pain? Fever? Low PaO_2 *and* high respiratory rate indicates cardiac or respiratory problem
● RR >30 per min (trend increasing)	**Becoming critical** Check gases for signs of respiratory failure
● RR reduced	**Could be critical** Oversedation? Neurological incident? Fatigue? Check gases for signs of respiratory failure
Work of breathing	Use of accessories and pursed lipped breathing may suggest fatigue
Breathing pattern	Irregular breathing pattern may be linked to fatigue or neurological damage

Table 3.7 *Continued*

Observations	Relevance
Expansion	Is it equal? Decreased movement may be linked to **loss of lung volume** (see Chapter 7)
Oxygen therapy	Take into account any oxygen patient is receiving when interpreting SaO_2/PaO_2. Is current therapy adequate? Hypoxaemia is classified as inability to keep PaO_2 above 8 kPa. See Chapter 9
Pulse oximetry (SpO_2) ● Normal range 95–98%	Look for trends and report any deterioration (sats of 90% may be less worrying than sats that have dropped from 98% to 92%) *In acute illness* – Below 92% may be significant *but* expect slightly lower values in elderly patients and during sleep *Patients with reduced cardiac output* – Slight hypoxaemia below 94% may be significant – Patients who are peripherally shut down may not have adequate blood flow to detect saturations; check trace! *Chronic chest patient* – Hypoxaemia may not be significant for chronic patients until below 80–85%. Compare with 'usual' values for patient (does the team have any accepted parameters?)
Arterial blood gases	Use a systematic approach to look at gases to identify a patient in (or developing) respiratory failure (see Fig. 3.2 and Chapter 9)
Chest X-rays	Is there any indication of specific problems? Are there any changes? See Table 3.8 for a system for interpretation
Cough	Is cough effective and is patient at risk of **sputum retention**?
Sputum	Viscosity, colour, smell, volume, presence of haemoptysis. How easy is it to clear and is there a risk of **sputum retention**?
Chest shape	Chest wall defects will **reduce lung volumes** and predispose the patient to **increased work of breathing**
Hands	Peripheral cyanosis, clubbing, temperature, nicotine stains. Is this a **chronic** problem?
Surgical wounds	Consider site and procedure the patient may have undergone (see Chapters 13 and 15). **Pain** from the wound and the anaesthetic can **reduce lung volumes** and lead to **sputum retention**

Table 3.7 *Continued*

Observations	Relevance
Intercostal drains	Are they present, draining, bubbling or swinging? (see Chapter 15). Consider the effects of pain and immobility
Hb ● 12–18 g/100 ml	High values suggest polycythaemia Low values suggest anaemia Consider before interpreting SpO_2 as affects oxygen content. (A patient with low saturations may have normal oxygen content if haemoglobin levels are very high)

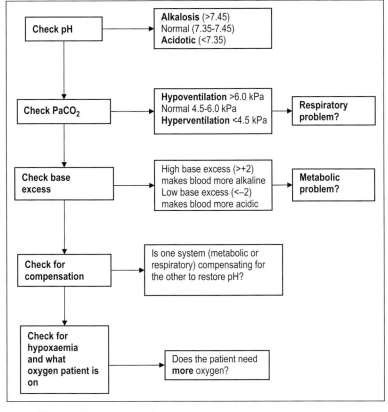

Figure 3.2 Arterial blood gas analysis.

Table 3.8 A system for chest X-ray interpretation – questions to ask

Keeping the film in context	About the film itself	
WHO – is the film of?	**A** – Alignment and A quick look	Is it a straight film? Is there anything obvious that jumps out?
WHAT – was taken?	**B** – Bones	Are they all there and intact?
WHERE – was it taken?	**C** – Cardiac	Is it in the correct position, the right size and has clear borders?
WHEN – was it taken?	**D** – Diaphragms	Are they in the correct position; are there clear contours and angles?
WHY – was it taken?	**E** – Expansion and Extra-thoracic structures	Is the chest well expanded? Examine structures outside the thorax
HOW – was it taken?	**F** – lung Fields	Are the lung fields clear and do they extend to the edge of the thorax?
	G – Gadgets	Are there any lines, drains, tubes, sutures, clips, etc.?

See Chapter 5 for more details on CXRs. As with ABGs, taking a systematic approach to reviewing data means that you are less likely to miss something. This is one system; if you use another and are happy using it, continue to do so.

Use the above A–G method to review the chest X-ray in Figure 3.3. This is a routine PA film of a 29-year-old female.
  Is it normal?

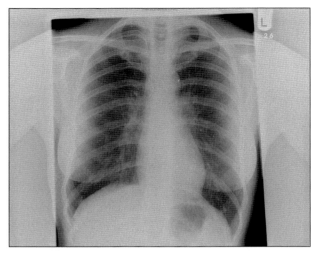

Figure 3.3 Chest X-ray of a 29-year-old female.

PHYSICAL EXAMINATION

Surface anatomy/surface marking

A sound knowledge of normal surface anatomy will facilitate your assessment. The guidance in Fig. 3.4 is for normal adults. Pathologies will lead to changes in anatomy and you must adapt your assessment as appropriate.

Palpation

Consider the elements in Tables 3.9 and 3.10.

Table 3.9 Palpation

Temperature	How hot/cold does the patient feel. Compare central to peripheral
Oedema	Is there any obvious central or peripheral oedema. See Cardiovascular section. If so, how might this impact on the treatment?
Trachea	Is it central? If not, do you feel it has been pushed to one side, for example by a mass or pulled over by collapse? Is this a new finding?
Expansion	Is it equal and is this maintained throughout the inspiratory and expiratory cycle?
Tactile fremitus	Can you feel any crackles under your hands? Use this to guide later aspects of the examination, in terms of percussion note and auscultation

Anterior view		
The apex of the lung 2 cm above the mid-point of the clavicle	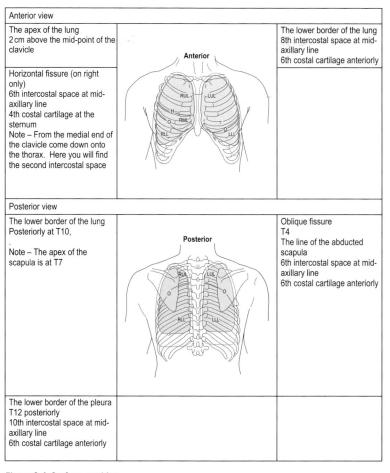 **Anterior**	The lower border of the lung 8th intercostal space at mid-axillary line 6th costal cartilage anteriorly
Horizontal fissure (on right only) 6th intercostal space at mid-axillary line 4th costal cartilage at the sternum Note – From the medial end of the clavicle come down onto the thorax. Here you will find the second intercostal space		
Posterior view		
The lower border of the lung Posteriorly at T10, . Note – The apex of the scapula is at T7	**Posterior**	Oblique fissure T4 The line of the abducted scapula 6th intercostal space at mid-axillary line 6th costal cartilage anteriorly
The lower border of the pleura T12 posteriorly 10th intercostal space at mid-axillary line 6th costal cartilage anteriorly		

Figure 3.4 Surface marking.

Table 3.10 Percussion note

Performed by placing a finger horizontally on the chest wall between two ribs and tapping sharply with a finger of the other hand	
Resonant due to air in thorax	● Air in lung (normal)
Hyperresonant	● Air between the pleura (pneumothorax) ● Overexpanded lung (emphysema)
A dull sound and flat feel due to fluid or solid	● Normal over liver or abdominal contents ● Pleural effusion ● Consolidation

AUSCULTATION

This includes breath sounds and added sounds (Tables 3.11–3.14).

Table 3.11 Breath sounds

Normal breath sounds ● Soft, muffled, louder on inspiration, fade in expiration, ratio 1:2	Turbulence in the large airways
Bronchial breathing ● Expiration louder and longer with pause between inspiration and expiration (like Darth Vader) ● Heard normally over trachea	If heard over lung fields, suggests: ● Consolidation ● Collapse without a plug ● May also be heard at the lip of a pleural effusion
Breath sounds quiet or absent? ● Poor air entry ● Low lung volumes ● Atelectasis	May be due to: ● Shallow breathing ● Poor positioning ● Collapse with complete obstruction of airway ● Sounds filtered by air (hyperinflation) ● Sounds filtered by pleura, chest wall (obese or muscular patients, pleural effusion, haemothorax) ● Pneumothorax
HAZARD: If you auscultate and hear a 'silent' chest, it may mean the patient is in extremis and is unable to move air at all (check airway and stethoscope). This is a medical emergency and you need to seek expert medical assistance straight away	

Table 3.12 Added sounds: crackles (short, non-musical popping sounds, fine or coarse)

Crackles	Cause and clinical relevance	
Fine crackles ● Reopening of airways sounds like rubbing hair next to your ear	● Atelectasis	● Short, explosive ● Periphery of lung ● Reduce with deep breath
	● Intra-alveolar oedema	● 'Tissue paper' ● Do not resolve with deep breath or cough ● Late inspiration (NB: interstitial fibrosis)
	● Secretions – small airways	● High pitched ● Peripheral ● Clear with cough
Coarse crackles ● Sounds like pouring milk on rice krispies	Obstruction more proximal and larger airways with sputum. May be inspiratory as well as expiratory	● Early expiratory – central airways ● Late expiratory – more peripheral airways ● Large deep sound ● Changes/clears with coughing

Remember, crackles are only heard if velocity of airflow is adequate and breath sounds audible!

Table 3.13 Added sounds: wheezes

Wheezes	Musical sounds due to vibration of wall of narrowed airway	
High-pitched wheeze	Bronchospasm	● Potential increased work of breathing
Low-pitched wheeze	Sputum	● Disrupted turbulent flow ● Change with coughing
Localized wheeze	Tumour Foreign body	● Limited to a local area on auscultation

Table 3.14 Other sounds

	Sounds like	Cause
Pleural rub	● Creaking/rubbing (like boots on snow) ● Localized/generalized ● Soft/loud ● Equal inspiration to expiration	● Inflammation of pleura ● Infection ● Tumour
Stridor	● Constant pitch on inspiration and expiration ● Produced in upper airways	● Croup ● Laryngeal tumour ● Upper airway obstruction **Alert medical staff** as the patient's airway is at great risk of compromise!

EARLY WARNING SCORES

The aim of these scores is two-fold:

1. To highlight changes in the physiological status of the patient with routine observations.
2. To empower staff to act and seek additional support for patients whose status has deteriorated (Table 3.15).

A significant change in the score (of 3 in one or more categories, or 3 and over in total depending on the scoring system) can trigger outreach or critical care support – see local policy for referral.

If the patient has not reached the trigger score – this does *not* preclude a call for help or advice.

THINGS CHANGE!

A patient may improve or deteriorate during your assessment/treatment and this does not necessarily reflect badly on your treatment. You may need to go back to the beginning again (ABC) to ensure patient safety.

Table 3.15 An example of an early warning score (Morgan et al. 1997, Subbe et al. 2001)

Score	3	2	1	0	1	2	3
Heart rate (HR)		<40	41–50	51–100	101–110	111–130	>130
Blood pressure (BP) (systolic)	<70	71–80	81–100	101–179	180–199	200–220	>220
Respiratory rate per minute		<8	8–11	12–20	21–25	26–30	>30
Total urine output in last 4 hours (ml)	<80	80–120	120–200		>800		
Central nervous system			Confusion	Awake/responsive	responding to Voice	responding to Pain	Unresponsive
Oxygen saturations	<85%	86–89%	90–94%	>95%			
Respiratory support/ oxygen therapy	NIV/CPAP	>10 litres/min oxygen	Oxygen therapy				

POTENTIAL PROBLEM LIST

Throughout this chapter an effort has been made to relate clinical findings to patient problems. At this stage of the assessment you should have a clear idea of what physiotherapy problems the patient has.

- Sputum retention?   see Chapter 6
- Decreased lung volume?   see Chapter 7
- Increased work of breathing?   see Chapter 8
- Respiratory failure?   see Chapter 9

CXR answer: This is a normal chest X-ray.

References

Morgan RJM, Williams F, Wright MM (1997) An early warning scoring system for detecting developing critical illness. Clinical Intensive Care 8:100.

Subbe CP, Kruger M, Rutherford P, Gemmell L (2001) Validation of a modified early warning score in medical admissions. Quarterly Journal of Medicine 94:521–6.

Acknowledgement

The editors would like to acknowledge the contribution of Hazel Horobin MCSP as author of the Assessment chapter in the first edition of this text.

CHAPTER 4

Paediatric specifics

Fiona Roberts

Although children develop the same respiratory problems they are not miniature adults. Age alters anatomy and physiology predisposing children to respiratory complications. Any intervention must be adapted to accommodate these changes. The differences are highlighted in this chapter.

CONSENT

● A legal requirement
● Children under 16 years of age can give consent if they fully understand what is involved – Gillick Competence (Chartered Society of Physiotherapy 2005)
● Refusal of treatment can be overridden by an adult with parental responsibility
● This also applies to 16 and 17 year olds *except* in Scotland where a person aged 16 and over is deemed an adult and the usual conditions for consent apply
● An adult with parental responsibility can give consent if the child is unable to do so
● If an emergency arises and the child is unable to give consent and/or someone with parental responsibility is unavailable it is

    '. . . acceptable to undertake treatment to preserve life or prevent serious damage to health'

                                                                              DoH (2001)

● Children sometimes refuse consent because they are frightened or do not understand.

CHILD PROTECTION

All physiotherapists who may be required to treat a child should know how to access information regarding child protection and how to raise any concerns they may have.

COMMUNICATING WITH A CHILD

When assessing a child:

- Remember they may be very frightened, which can result in poor compliance.
- Use language appropriate to their stage of development.
- Persuasion may be necessary.
- Play, distraction and/or rewards may enhance compliance.
- Involving parents may help; ask them to demonstrate, coax, explain, etc.

PARENTS

- If they are present parents will be very concerned, anxious and possibly frightened.
- These emotions can manifest themselves in many different ways.
- Always remember this if parents react in an unexpected way.
- Use tact and understanding with them.
- Always explain who you are and what you are going to do in a way that they will understand.

ANATOMICAL AND PHYSIOLOGICAL DIFFERENCES IN CHILDREN

Anatomical and physiological differences resolve as children age but have significant influence on respiratory problems particularly in children less than 5 years of age. Tables 4.1 and 4.2 detail the differences and their clinical implications.

RESPONSE TO HYPOXAEMIA

- Infants have higher basal metabolic rates than adults which results in higher oxygen consumption rates and greater demand for oxygen.
- Hypoxia can, therefore, develop rapidly.
- Infants' response to hypoxia is to drop their heart rate to below 100 beats per minute (b.p.m.) (bradycardia).
- This can trigger pulmonary vasoconstriction, which worsens the oxygenation status by limiting blood flow through the lungs.

THORACIC DIFFERENCES

The first four points in Table 4.1 prevent young children from increasing tidal volume (TV) to increase minute volume (MV).

- Respiratory rate is increased to achieve this
- Causes increased respiratory muscle work
- Fatigue likely.

Table 4.1 Thoracic differences

Difference	Effect	Clinical implications
Ribs more horizontal in infants	No bucket handle effect	● Cannot increase depth of breath
Rib cage more compliant due to immature bone formation (rigidity increases as child reaches 8 years of age)	Less thoracic stability	● When respiratory load increases, pressure changes result in indrawing of soft tissue, i.e. recession (Table 4.3) ● When positioning, underlying lung may be compressed and compromised ● May make manual techniques more effective ● Possible risk of atelectasis due to vibrations reducing functional residual capacity (FRC)
Respiratory muscles contain fewer slow-twitch fibres – adult 55%, child 30%	Muscles will fatigue more quickly	● Very limited respiratory reserve ● Respiratory fatigue develops very rapidly ● Prompt and appropriate intervention required to prevent distress developing into fatigue
Intercostal muscles lack tone, power, coordination	Unable to provide significant assistance when respiratory load increases Do not help provide thoracic stability	● Intercostal recession results (Table 4.3)
Heart : lung ratio relatively larger in infants, i.e. 1 : 1 compared to $\frac{1}{3}$: $\frac{2}{3}$ in adults	Less space for lungs	● If heart size increases lungs will be compromised ● This will influence positioning – may not tolerate supine or side lying

4

Table 4.2 Airway differences

Difference	Effect	Clinical implications
Infants and babies have relatively larger tongues, tonsils and adenoids in comparison with adults	Predominantly nose breathers	● If nose obstructed with secretions work of breathing can increase (nasogastric tubes – NGT – can have same effect)
Small airway diameter Infant trachea 5–6 mm Adult trachea 14–15 mm	Increases resistance to airflow	● Small changes in airway diameter significantly increase resistance ● Obstruction occurs more easily which will increase work of breathing, reduce lung volumes
Trachea's narrowest point: cricoid cartilage	Unable to use cuffed endotracheal tube (ETT) – will cause damage	● Uncuffed ETT used ● Difficult to secure – extreme care required not to dislodge ETT ● Bypassing of secretions up sides of ETT ● Also risk of vomit and oral secretions reaching lungs ● Any trauma will lead to significant oedema and airway obstruction (see below – stridor)
Floppy cartilage in trachea	Poor airway support	● Predisposed to airway collapse ● **! Bronchodilators can worsen this. Use with caution**
Immature cilia	Reduced efficiency of mucociliary transport	● Risk of infection ● Reduced ability to cope with increased secretion quantity ● Increased risk of retained secretions and airway collapse
Fewer, smaller alveoli (increase in numbers until 10–12 years then increase in size only)	Reduced gas exchange area	● Small amount of collapse/ consolidation can cause significant changes in respiratory status, e.g. hypoxaemia, increased work of breathing
Absent pores of Kohn and canals of Lambert until approx. 5 years of age	No collateral ventilation	● Cannot use collateral ventilation to help re-inflate collapse

Helpful Hint

Prone positioning provides thoracic stability and facilitates diaphragm function.

! Due to sudden infant death syndrome, babies who are not constantly supervised should not be left in prone position without monitoring, e.g. apnoea alarm, pulse oximeter.

AIRWAY DIFFERENCES

! Stridor (narrowing of upper trachea and/or larynx, usually heard on inspiration) can be caused by: trauma, infection, foreign body or congenital problems.

Do not treat unless origin is known and physiotherapy will not worsen condition.

Summary
- More prone to atelectasis and retained secretions
- Will fatigue quickly
- Deterioration (and improvement) can be rapid.

OTHER DIFFERENCES

Older children usually demonstrate the same signs of respiratory distress as adults (see Chapter 3).

Signs of respiratory distress seen in young children and babies are shown in Table 4.3.

All signs may not be seen together.

Handy Hint

Babies/children with chronic respiratory problems normally show some of these signs (Table 4.3). It is important to compare their current signs with normal, to identify whether you should be concerned.

Table 4.3 Signs of respiratory distress

Sign	Cause	Other information
Increased respiratory rate	Required to increase minute volume	● Age dependent
Recession: – subcostal – intercostal – sternal – suprasternal (tracheal tug) – supraclavicular	Identified areas sucked inwards during inspiratory pressure change due to lack of thoracic stability/ muscle tone	● Mild/moderate/severe grades ● Seen in babies, young children and those unable to fix their thoracic cage
Head bobbing	Attempt to use accessory respiratory muscles but unable to fix	● Sometimes seen as rotation if supine
Nasal flare	Primitive response to entrain more air	● No actual effect
Expiratory grunting (auto PEEP)	Trying to increase intrinsic positive end expiratory pressure (PEEP) and reduce work of breathing	● Increases FRC ● Severe if audible at bedside ● Less severe if only audible with stethoscope
See-sawing	Forceful contraction of diaphragm Causes abdomen to be pushed out and generates massive negative pressure in thorax, sucking chest wall in	● **! Unsustainable** ● **If observed immediate intervention required** ● **Call medical staff**
Neck extension	Trying to reduce airflow resistance to reduce work of breathing	● In intubated children can be an attempt to get away from ETT ● Could also be due to abnormal tone ● Determine cause to enable appropriate intervention
Apnoea	Temporary cessation of breathing	● **Child is fatiguing and requires urgent respiratory support and/ or stimulation**

Table 4.4 Additional subjective information from medical notes

Information required	Clinical relevance
Birth history: – Was child born prematurely? – Postnatal problems? – Ventilation? – Lung condition?	● Preterm babies may have chronic lung conditions, e.g. bronchopulmonary dysplasia (BPD), which cause poor lung compliance and impair gas exchange ● May normally have: recession, long-term oxygen therapy (LTOT), secretions, raised CO_2, increased respiratory rate (RR) ● BPD babies often do not tolerate handling ● Respond with desaturation, bradycardia, apnoea ● Prone to further respiratory problems, mainly during first year–18 months of life ● Little respiratory reserve so fatigue rapidly ● Need to be cautious using continuous positive airway pressure (CPAP)

Any history of intraventricular haemorrhage, periventricular leukomalacia, encephalopathies or birth trauma?	● Can manifest as altered neurological status causing abnormal muscle tone, posture or patterns of movement resulting in delayed or abnormal development
	● Additional problems that can result from altered neurological status:
	  – Poor cough
	  – Impaired swallow
	  – Poor airway protection
	● Can result in secretion problems and airway obstruction
	● May need to consider suction or tracheal rub only if you have been assessed in its use)

Pre-existing conditions	● Significant chest or spinal deformities can alter lung mechanics ● Some conditions result in respiratory muscle weakness, e.g. muscular dystrophy and spinal muscular atrophy ● Predisposes to respiratory complications and can also result in ineffective cough ● Problems with positioning, may need to use support, e.g. pillows or child's own postural management system
Any history of gastro-oesophageal reflux (GOR)	● If diagnosed, position with head up to prevent aspiration ● Recurrent chest problems may be due to GOR

4

Cyanosis (blue discoloration to mucous membranes) is an unreliable sign of hypoxaemia in babies and infants due to the amount and type of haemoglobin in their blood.

Handy Hint
No significant respiratory problem if: child sitting up/chatting/playing or a baby is able to take a bottle.
  ! If completely focused on breathing, e.g. uninterested in surroundings or stimuli, there is significant respiratory failure and prompt action is required.

ASSESSMENT
When assessing children we use all the information discussed in Chapter 3 and some specific to paediatrics (Tables 4.4 and 4.5). Some subjective information may be gained from the child, if you can ask them directly, or the parents/carer.

OBJECTIVE INFORMATION
Tables 4.6 and 4.7 show those factors with special significance in the assessment of children.

AUSCULTATION
There are several issues to consider when using auscultation on a child (Table 4.8).

COMMON CONDITIONS
Table 4.9 is a list of common conditions referred for on call physiotherapy and the implications they have for assessment.

Helpful Hint
If suspected NAI:
Ensure you document any fractures identified from CXR
Remember your role is to treat the baby/child – not judge

Table 4.5 Other subjective information specific to children

Information	Clinical relevance

Tolerance of handling:
● Do they desaturate?
● How quickly and to what level?
● Speed of recovery?
● Do they become bradycardic?
● Self-resolving or requiring stimulation to resolve?
● When were they last handled?
● Recovery time?
	● Usually indicate:
	  – How sick the child is – commonly sicker children handle badly, e.g. desaturate, become bradycardic
	  – Degree of oxygen dependency
	● If handled recently and responded badly, consider rest period before any intervention
	● Implications for how much assessment and/or treatment will be tolerated
	● Consider incorporating recovery time into assessment/treatment

Social history including development	● If parents/carers present, who are you speaking to? ● Do they have parental responsibility? Consent? ● Relevant information: e.g. care orders, psychological issues with child ● Influence how you approach the child, e.g. level of communication ● What can the child do for you?
Feeds: ● Bottle-feeding/breast? ● Nasogastric tube feeding? Bolus or continuous? ● Feeds stopped?	● Inability to suck a bottle indicates SOB ● Abdominal distension impairs diaphragm function ● Continuous NG feeds/no feeds reduce diaphragmatic compromise ● Those with severe respiratory distress will be on continuous or no feed
If on bolus feeds when was last one?	● Leave intervention for at least an hour after feed to prevent vomiting
Signs of pain: ● Some children cannot express pain verbally. Look for other signs: ● Thumbs tucked in fist ● Frown ● Lethargy ● Irritability	● Be observant and aware of the possible signs ● Missing signs will cause more pain if moving/treating child ● Thumbs tucked in could be due to abnormal tone if underlying neurological problem ● Pain could cause increased tone and exaggeration of abnormal movement patterns or postures in those with neurological problems

4

Table 4.6 Objective factors

Objective finding	Change and clinical significance
Temperature	● Pyrexia can induce febrile convulsions in young children and babies ● Child will be very sleepy after fitting ● If baby pyrexial do not cover them up/obstruct fan ● Low temperature in a baby can increase oxygen requirements
CVS: Heart rate and blood pressure Bradycardia	● Normal values alter with age (see Chapter 3) ● Indicative of fatigue and/or hypoxaemia ● If not self-resolving may require stimulation (pat on the bottom, rub chest) and increased supplemental oxygen
Respiratory rate Apnoeas – more than 20 s between breaths	● Values change with age (see Appendix 2) ● Apnoeas can indicate respiratory distress, secretions or sepsis ● May require stimulation (as for bradycardia)
Oxygen saturation	● Same as adult unless treating: – Child with cyanotic cardiac defect (will have predetermined acceptable levels)
Oxygen device adequate?	● See Table 4.7

Endotracheal tubes (ETT)	● Children nasally intubated unless contraindicated (e.g. skull fracture)
	● Provides greater security for ETT
	● Predisposed to:
	  – Airway leaks
	  – Bypass of secretions

Tracheostomy	● Unusual in children: once removed tracheostomy site can cause tracheal stenosis
	● If present means:
	  – Long-term airway problems
	  – Very long-term ventilation

Fluid balance	● Children are much smaller; therefore smaller positive volumes can be significant for them ● Urine output usually 1–2 ml/kg/h ● Positive volume of 200 ml significant for a small baby, insignificant for an 8-year-old ● Large positive balance – makes secretions very loose/ causes pulmonary oedema ● Negative balance – could cause tenacious secretions

Table 4.7 Oxygen delivery devices

Device	Clinical implications
Masks	● Too big for babies ● Babies/infants often dislike masks
Blow/flow by	● Mask placed near baby's face ● Entrains large volume of air from environment with each breath, reduced oxygen content
Head box	● Plastic box with oxygen piped in. Placed over baby's head to provide an oxygen-rich environment ● Baby/infant may slide out towards opening for trunk ● Oxygen concentration then lower due to ambient air entrainment ● Carbon dioxide retention can occur if not suitably ventilated, e.g. baby too big for opening
Nasal prongs	● Can be used even on babies. Direct administration to airway but limited flow possible (2 litres/minute) (FiO_2 0.28)

Table 4.8 Auscultation

Issue	Clinical implication
Secretions pool in posterior lung areas, especially bases, due to prolonged periods in supine position	● Must listen to posterior aspect of thorax
Small distance between upper airways and lungs	● Transmitted sounds common ● Can be misleading ● Always listen without stethoscope first then compare sounds
Adult stethoscopes cover large areas of thorax	● Difficult to localize problem area
Upper lobe common site of collapse/consolidation	● Listen to upper zones anteriorly and posteriorly

Table 4.9 Common conditions

Condition	Implications for physiotherapy
Bronchiolitis	● Physiotherapy not recommended unless the child has required admission to ICU (probable superimposed infection) (SIGN 2006) ● If ventilated, assess carefully. If area of reduced air entry and/or crackles on auscultation, treat as appropriate as indicative of collapse and/or retained secretions ● Whether ventilated or not, these babies often desaturate with handling
Whooping cough (pertussis)	● Physiotherapy contraindicated in acute stages ● If ventilated, paralysed and sedated – treat if crackles indicating retained secretions or reduced air entry indicating focal collapse found on assessment
Croup (acute laryngotracheobronchitis)	● Physiotherapy contraindicated in the non-intubated child
Acute epiglottitis	● Physiotherapy contraindicated in the non-intubated child ● Only treat the intubated child if assessment indicates need
Pneumonia	● Manual techniques only effective if assessment indicates sputum retention (crackles on auscultation) ● Position for good ventilation/perfusion matching
Inhaled foreign body	● Only treat, if indicated, once foreign body removed
Non-accidental injury (NAI)	● If child admitted with concerns of NAI be aware of neurological complications, e.g. signs of fitting, Modified Glasgow Coma Score ● May have rib fractures

SUMMARY

- Children are prone to atelectasis and retained secretions
- Small areas of atelectasis or small amounts of secretion can cause significant deterioration in work of breathing and gas exchange
- Children have poor respiratory reserves
- If signs of respiratory distress (see Box 4.1) intervene quickly
- Bradycardia = hypoxia
- If child is playing, chatting, taking a bottle with no problems, there is no significant respiratory problem
- Adapt your approach to suit the child's development
- Keep parents informed

Box 4.1 Signs of respiratory distress

- Raised respiratory rate (dependent on age)
- Subcostal recession
- Intercostal recession
- Sternal recession
- Supraclavicular recession (tracheal tug)
- Head bobbing
- Nasal flare
- Grunting
- Apnoea

References

Chartered Society of Physiotherapy (2005) Consent. London: CSP.

Department of Health (2001) Seeking consent: working with children. London: HMSO.

SIGN (2006) Bronchiolitis in children. Guideline 91. Edinburgh: Scottish Intercollegiate Guidelines Network.

Further reading

Arthur R (2000) Interpretation of the paediatric chest x-ray. Paediatr Respir Rev 1:41–50.

Frownfelter D, Dean E (2006) Cardiovascular and pulmonary physical therapy. Evidence and practice, 4th edn, Chapter 37. St Louis: Mosby.

CHAPTER 5

Chest X-ray interpretation

Stephen Harden

The emphasis of this chapter is the X-ray appearance of common conditions that you will see when on call. As the majority of patients requiring emergency physiotherapy are short of breath or have suboptimal gas exchange, only abnormalities of the lungs and pleural spaces are demonstrated. Only frontal X-rays (posteroanterior (PA) and anteroposterior (AP)) are used as these are the ones that you will be required to interpret.

Remember that a perfect chest X-ray (CXR; Fig. 5.1) requires correct patient positioning and the correct X-ray dose. Deficiency in any of these results in a suboptimal X-ray and may produce appearances that simulate lung pathology.

NORMAL LOBAR ANATOMY

- The right lung contains three lobes, upper (RUL), middle (RML) and lower (RLL) (Fig. 5.2A, B).
- On the right side, the oblique fissure separates the RUL from the RLL above the horizontal fissure and the RML from the RLL below it.
- The horizontal fissure separates the RUL from the RML.

> **Remember**
> When looking at a frontal CXR:
> - RUL is at the top above the horizontal fissure
> - RML is at the base anteriorly below the horizontal fissure
> - RLL is posterior

- The left lung consists of two lobes, upper (LUL) and lower (LLL) (Fig. 5.2C). The lingula is the most inferior part of the LUL
- The oblique fissure on the left side separates the LUL and LLL

Figure 5.1 Normal chest X-ray. Key: 1, trachea; 2, horizontal fissure; 3, costophrenic angle; 4, right hemidiaphragm; 5, left hemidiaphragm; 6, heart shadow; 7, aortic arch; 8, right hilum; 9, left hilum.

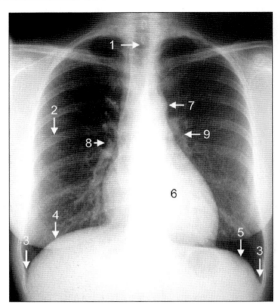

Remember

The LUL is anterior and the LLL is posterior.

For descriptive purposes, the lungs on the CXR are divided into thirds or zones (Fig. 5.2D):

- upper zone
- mid-zone
- lower zone.

These are *not* anatomical divisions. For example, the apex of the lower lobe on each side is in the mid-zone.

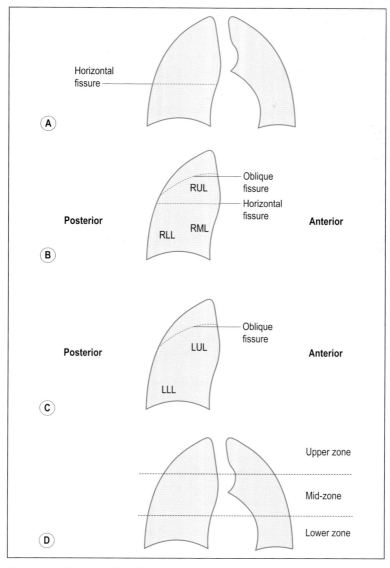

Figure 5.2 Fields on the CXR. (A) Frontal plane. (B) Right lung, lateral. (C) Left lung, lateral. (D) Lung field zones.

HOW TO INTERPRET ABNORMALITIES IN THE LUNG FIELDS ON THE CXR

Essentially, these areas are abnormal because they appear either:

● too white or
● too black.

Too white

The vast majority of abnormalities in the on call setting are areas that are too white and the commonest causes are:

● collapse or atelectasis
● consolidation
● pleural effusion
● pulmonary oedema.

Too black

When there are areas which appear too black, the most important causes are:

● pneumothorax
● COPD.

Each of these is described below.

ATELECTASIS/COLLAPSE

Atelectasis or collapse refers to an area of lung which is airless and the lung collapses in this region. Atelectasis may involve an entire lobe or even an entire lung.

The chest X-ray will show a loss of lung volume. This means that the lung field will be smaller than expected. Other structures may move to fill up the space, so there may be:

● shift of the mediastinal structures such as the heart or trachea
● elevation of the hemidiaphragm compared to the other side.

The area of collapsed lung appears as a white or 'dense' area and this represents airless lung tissue. When this affects a small volume of the lung, the appearance is of a white line and this is often seen at the lung bases in postoperative patients. When a whole lobe collapses, each produces a specific appearance (Table 5.1).

When a whole lung collapses there is increased density of the entire hemithorax (Figs 5.8 and 5.9). This appearance is sometimes called a 'white-out', although there are other causes for this. A pneumonectomy is in effect an extreme form of complete lung collapse and so will look the same on CXR but you may see rib irregularity marking the site of the thoracotomy.

Table 5.1 Appearance of lobar collapse

Lobe collapse	Presentation
RUL collapse	● There is increased density high in the right lung down to the horizontal fissure ● This fissure swings upwards and can adopt an almost vertical position (Fig. 5.3)
RML collapse	● The RML collapses down against the right heart border which becomes indistinct (Fig. 5.4) ● The right heart border is clearly seen on a normal CXR because it lies adjacent to the air-filled middle lobe
RLL collapse	● There is a triangular density low in the right lung but the right heart border can still be clearly seen (Fig. 5.5)
LUL collapse	● The left lung is slightly whiter than the right ● The LUL is anterior and so collapses against the anterior chest wall. Thus, you see air in the LLL through the dense collapsed LUL (Fig. 5.6)
LLL collapse	● A triangular density is seen behind the heart (Fig. 5.7) ● The part of the heart shadow to the left of the spine is whiter than that to the right of the spine

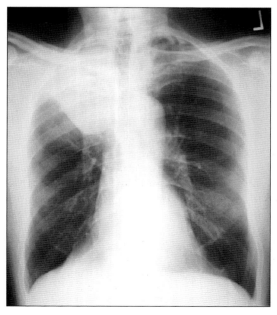

Figure 5.3 Right upper lobe collapse. The horizontal fissure is now oriented obliquely. The trachea is deviated to the right which is evidence of mediastinal shift.

Figure 5.4 Right middle lobe collapse. The right heart border is indistinct and there is a vague white appearance to the adjacent lung.

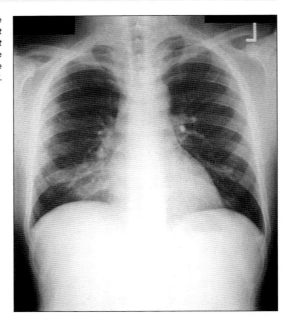

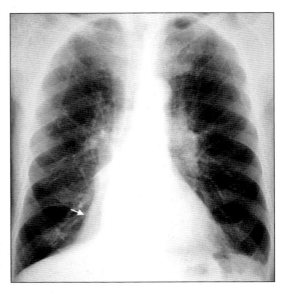

Figure 5.5 Right lower lobe collapse. There is abnormal whiteness with a straight outer border (arrow) low in the right lung. The right heart border is still visible.

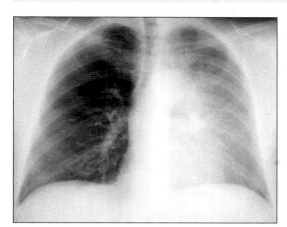

Figure 5.6 Left upper lobe collapse. There is a hazy increased whiteness over the left hemithorax. The left heart border is indistinct.

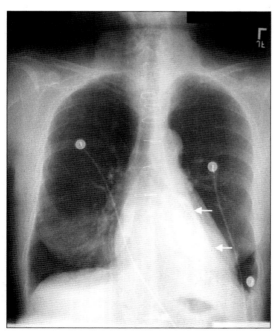

Figure 5.7 Left lower lobe collapse. Increased whiteness is seen behind the heart with a straight outer edge (arrows).

Figure 5.8 Left lung collapse. There is abnormal whiteness over the left hemithorax. The heart is shifted to the left within the abnormal area.

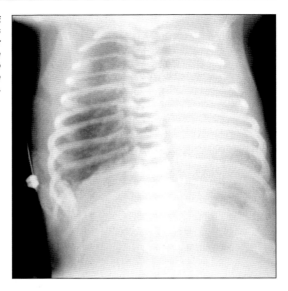

Figure 5.9 Pneumonectomy. Abnormal whiteness is seen in the left hemithorax. The trachea and heart are shifted to the left.

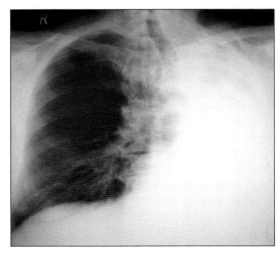

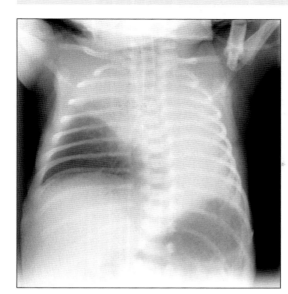

Figure 5.10 Collapse of the left lung and right upper lobe. Note the tip of the ET tube which lies in the right bronchus intermedius.

5

Remember

When you see complete collapse of the left lung associated with RUL collapse in a ventilated patient always check the position of the endotracheal tube. If the tube has been advanced down the right main bronchus then only the RML and RLL will be aerated (Fig. 5.10).

CONSOLIDATION

Consolidation occurs when air in lung is replaced by fluid. The distribution of this consolidation may be patchy or may affect an entire segment or lobe. The composition of this fluid depends on the cause:

● infected fluid, as in pneumonia (the commonest cause that you will see)
● saliva or gastric contents, seen in cases of aspiration
● blood, in cases of traumatic lung contusion
● serous transudate, seen in alveolar pulmonary oedema.

Although the distribution may help to elicit the cause, the radiological appearance of consolidation is the same for all of these.

Radiological appearance

- The **whiteness or shadowing** in the lung is **poorly defined**. It is difficult to see the edges of these areas. The shadowing has been described as 'fluffy' in appearance.
- There is **no loss of volume,** unlike atelectasis, as there is no lung collapse (Fig. 5.11).
- An air **bronchogram** may be seen, particularly when there is extensive consolidation. This is caused by consolidation of lung tissue adjacent to an air-filled bronchus which thus stands out as a black tube amid the consolidative shadowing (Fig. 5.12).

Knowledge of lobar anatomy helps to localize consolidation as it does with atelectasis (Fig. 5.13). It is important in terms of how you treat your patient and may also provide clues as to the cause:

- Aspiration tends particularly to affect the right lower lobe when the patient is erect as the right main and lower lobe bronchi are the most vertical (Fig. 5.14).

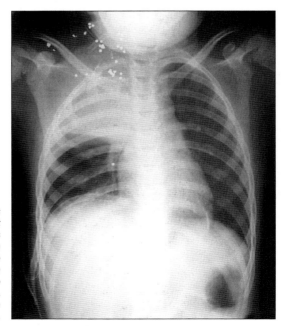

Figure 5.11 Traumatic consolidation of the right upper lobe. There is abnormal whiteness in the right upper lobe. The horizontal fissure is in its normal position, so there is no volume loss. Note the shrapnel in the soft tissues.

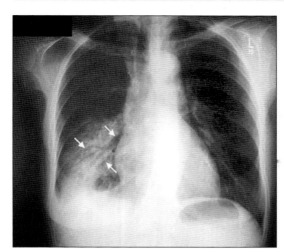

Figure 5.12 Right lower lobe consolidation. The abnormal whiteness in the right lower and mid-zones is poorly defined and 'fluffy'. There is a trident-shaped lucency which is an air bronchogram (arrows). The right heart border remains visible.

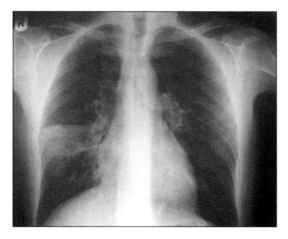

Figure 5.13 Middle lobe consolidation. The poorly defined 'fluffy' increased whiteness abuts the horizontal fissure and there is no volume loss.

- Aspiration is particularly seen in the apical segments of the lower lobes when the patient is supine as these bronchi are directed posteriorly and are thus the most dependent in a patient lying flat.
- Lung contusion tends to occur in the setting of trauma so there may be skin bruising and you may see rib fractures on the CXR (Fig. 5.15).
- In alveolar pulmonary oedema, the consolidation appearance tends to be situated in the mid-zones around the hila.

5

Figure 5.14 Right lower lobe consolidation. The upper limit of this abnormal whiteness shows the location of the apical segment of the right lower lobe, which is in the mid-zone.

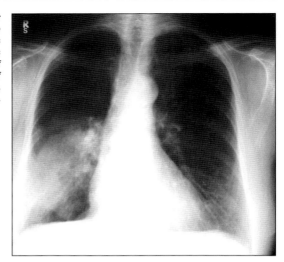

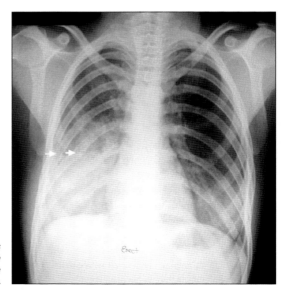

Figure 5.15 Traumatic right lower lobe consolidation. Note the rib fractures (arrows).

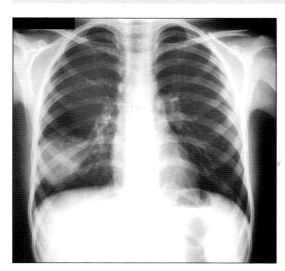

Figure 5.16 Round pneumonia. The rounded patchy white area in the right lower zone represents consolidation.

In children, infective consolidation is often circular in shape. This is termed a round pneumonia (Fig. 5.16).

> **Remember**
> In real life, consolidation and atelectasis commonly occur together, but by analysing the abnormal white areas on the CXR you will find that one of these tends to predominate and thus is probably the most important when it comes to treating the patient.

PLEURAL EFFUSION

This refers to fluid in the pleural space. It occupies the dependent part of the pleural space due to gravity so when the patient is erect or semi-erect it occupies the lower zone on CXR initially. However, if the patient is supine, it occupies the posterior surface of the pleural space.

Radiological appearance

The characteristic feature of the abnormal whiteness of a pleural effusion is that its density is **uniform** throughout. It is not patchy.

Most patients that you will see will have their X-rays taken erect or semi-erect:

- A small effusion presents as blunting of the costophrenic angle, the region on the CXR between the hemidiaphragm and the chest wall.
- In a moderate-sized effusion, the top of the fluid is seen as a horizontal line and there is a meniscus at the point where the fluid touches the chest wall. The hemidiaphragm is obscured (Fig. 5.17).
- With a very large effusion there may be shift of the mediastinum away from the side of the effusion. A large effusion is another cause for a 'white-out' appearance but the position of the mediastinum tells you if it is due to atelectasis or effusion (Fig. 5.18).

If the patient is supine the fluid adopts a posterior location. Thus there will be a generalized increased whiteness of the lung field. The lung can still be seen and is effectively being viewed through a thin layer of fluid.

PULMONARY OEDEMA

The majority of cases are due to left ventricular failure. The features are:

- The heart is usually enlarged.
- There may be consolidation around the hila as described above (Fig. 5.19).

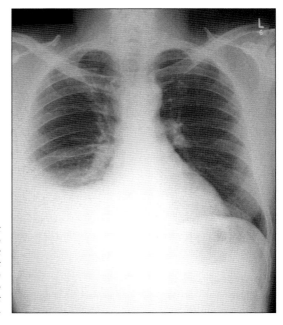

Figure 5.17 Right pleural effusion. There is uniform whiteness at the base of the right hemithorax with a horizontal upper surface and a meniscus seen at the chest wall.

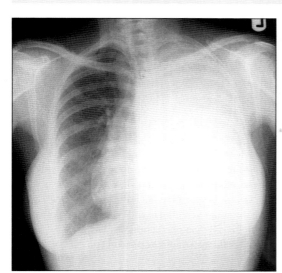

Figure 5.18 Left pleural effusion. There is uniform whiteness over the left hemithorax and the heart and mediastinum are displaced to the right. Thus there is 'too much volume' on the left due to a massive pleural effusion.

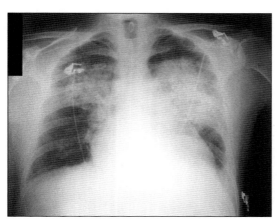

Figure 5.19 Heart failure and alveolar pulmonary oedema. The heart is enlarged and there is bilateral consolidation around the hila, the so-called 'bat's wing' appearance. Note the small left pleural effusion.

- There may be tiny, thin, horizontal lines which are seen in the lower zones where the lung touches the chest wall. These are due to oedema in the lung substance or interstitium rather than the alveoli and are known as Kerley B lines (Figs 5.20 and 5.21).
- There are large distended veins seen in the upper zones (Fig. 5.20).
- There may be pleural effusions.

PNEUMOTHORAX

This is an important cause of a lung field appearing *too black* and refers to air in the pleural space. The features on the CXR are:

- The lung edge is seen as a white line parallel to the chest wall (Fig. 5.22).
- Lung markings do not extend out beyond this white line.
- The area outside this lung edge is blacker than the area inside the line.

A pneumothorax may involve the entire hemithorax and in this case there will be no lung markings visible at all. In a tension pneumothorax the air in the pleural space steadily increases and can build up significant pressure, pushing the medi-

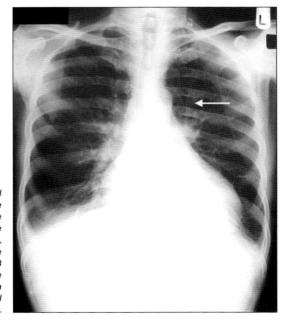

Figure 5.20 Interstitial pulmonary oedema. The heart is enlarged. There is prominence of the upper lobe veins (arrow), representing upper lobe blood diversion. Kerley B lines are seen at the right base and there is a small right-sided pleural effusion.

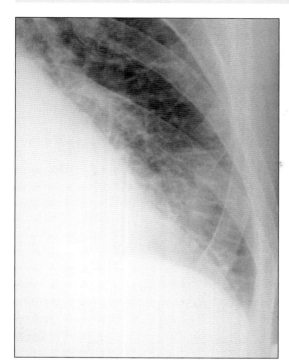

Figure 5.21 Kerley B lines. Thin horizontal white lines are seen reaching the pleural surface at the costophrenic angle.

astinum away towards the opposite side (Fig. 5.23). This can cause cardiac arrest and is thus a surgical emergency.

Hazard

You should not use positive pressure ventilation (e.g. CPAP, IPPB or NIV) in a patient with a pneumothorax as you may turn it into a tension pneumothorax.

Occasionally, the air in the pleural cavity may be located anteriorly, particularly when the patient is supine. This makes it more difficult to see as there may not be a visible lung edge. Be suspicious if the CXR of a ventilated patient shows one lung to be blacker than the other, particularly in the lower zone, and is associated with otherwise unexplained suboptimal gas exchange.

Figure 5.22 Right pneumothorax. A black area in the right hemithorax surrounds the right lung, whose edge is clearly seen as a white line (arrows). Lung markings do not extend into this black area.

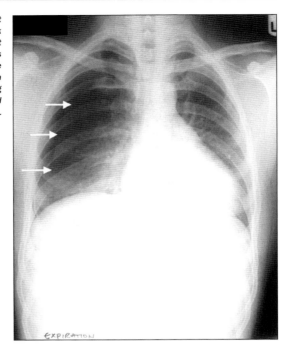

Figure 5.23 Left tension pneumothorax. The left hemithorax contains no lung markings at all. The heart and mediastinum are shifted to the right.

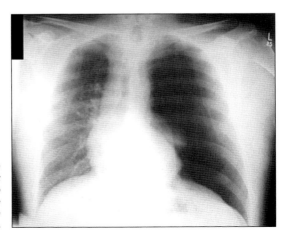

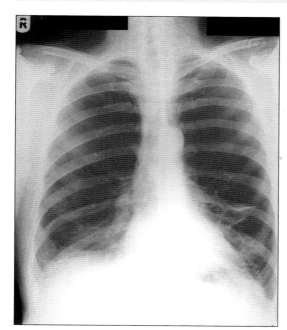

Figure 5.24 COPD. Both lungs are blacker than normal, particularly in the upper zones. No lung edge is visible. Close inspection shows lung markings reaching all the way to the pleural surface and chest wall on each side.

COPD

The lungs appear hyperinflated and blacker in emphysema due to the destruction of lung tissue. Thin-walled sacs or bullae may develop and appear as particularly black areas, often at the top of the lung. In these cases, unlike pneumothorax, there is no visible lung edge and lung markings are seen reaching the chest wall (Fig. 5.24).

Hazard

If you use positive pressure ventilation in these patients, be aware that there is a risk of creating a pneumothorax by rupturing one of the thin-walled bullae. Usually the benefits to the patient outweigh this small risk but it is important to discuss this with a doctor.

This chapter is a guide to help you interpret abnormal CXRs when on call. However, it is important to develop a systematic approach to reading a CXR so as to obtain all the information available to you.

! FLAG Refer to Chapter 3.

Acknowledgements

I am grateful to Dr D.J. Delany and Dr I.W. Brown for the use of their extensive film collection and to Dr J.D. Argent for supplying the film of round pneumonia.

Further reading

Corne J, Carroll M, Brown I, Delany D (2002) Chest X-ray made easy, 2nd edn. London: Churchill Livingstone.

CHAPTER 6

The management of sputum retention

Ruth Wakeman

This chapter considers the causes of sputum retention and offers suggestions for effective, appropriate treatment.

CLINICAL SIGNS OF SPUTUM RETENTION

See Table 6.1.

POTENTIAL CAUSES OF SPUTUM RETENTION

See Figure 6.1.

Table 6.1 Clinical signs of sputum retention

Patient	Clinical signs of sputum retention
Adult	● Increased work of breathing ● Auscultation: crackles (particularly on inspiration); wheeze; reduced or absent breath sounds ● Secretions: audible at the mouth or palpable through the chest wall ● Audible secretions or coarse wheeze on cough/huff ● ↓Oxygen saturations or PaO_2 (hypoxaemia) ● ↑$PaCO_2$ (hypercapnia) ● CXR shows patchy shadowing or atelectasis ● Infection: a. ↑Temperature b. ↑HR (tachycardia) c. Elevated inflammatory markers, i.e. white cell count (WCC) ● Patients may describe difficulty clearing secretions with associated clinical deterioration ● Possible associated tachycardia, restlessness, or cyanosis

Table 6.1 *Continued*

Patient	Clinical signs of sputum retention
Ventilated patients (in addition to those above):	● ↑Airway pressures if ventilated in volume control modes ● ↓Tidal volumes if pressure control modes (consider alternative reasons for these changes) ● Secretions on suction, with associated clinical deterioration. Alternatively secretions may be difficult to access ● Occlusion of the airway lumen may prevent introduction of a suction catheter
Child	● See adult section
Additionally:	● Age-related signs of increased work of breathing (Ch. 8) ● CXR – lobar collapse may be more common than in adults ● Coughing on exercise reported by children or carers
Ventilated children	● Increased peak inspiratory pressure requirements or a reduction in tidal volumes may be noted
Baby	● See adult section

Additionally:	● ↑Respiratory distress, e.g. common symptoms:
	  a. Subcostal, intercostal or sternal recession
	  b. Nasal flaring
	  c. Increased respiratory rate
	  d. Stridor
	  e. Cyanosis
	  f. Neck extension
	  g. Expiratory grunting
	  h. Tracheal tug
	● CXR – areas of collapse are relatively common with sputum retention

Ventilated babies	● As in children ● Diminished chest wall movement or 'wiggle' if high-frequency oscillatory ventilation is used
NB: The patient may present with one or more of the signs listed.	

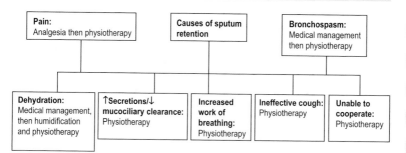

Figure 6.1 Potential causes of sputum retention.

EXCESSIVE SECRETIONS +/− IMPAIRED MUCOCILIARY CLEARANCE (Table 6.2)

Table 6.2 Treatments and suggested modifications for excessive secretions

Suggested treatment options/modifications	
Adult	
Active cycle of breathing (ACBT)	● Simple, easily modified, incorporating thoracic expansion exercises (TEEs), forced expiration technique (FET) and breathing control
Gravity-assisted positioning (GAP)	● Modify positioning where poorly tolerated. If mucociliary clearance is impaired (e.g. in primary ciliary dyskinesia) GAP may be important treatment choice
Manual techniques (MT)	● Chest percussion and shaking on expiration may aid sputum clearance

Table 6.2 *Continued*

Suggested treatment options/modifications	
Other treatment modalities	● Patients may already use other techniques, e.g. positive expiratory pressure (PEP), Flutter VRP1, Autogenic Drainage or RC Cornet™. It is not appropriate to start a new technique in the on call setting unless you are skilled in its use
Exercise	● Use exercise where tolerated; this complements other airway clearance techniques. Exercise may cause either bronchodilation or bronchoconstriction
Humidification	● Humidify oxygen if at all possible
IPPB	● IPPB is particularly useful where fatigue or work of breathing limits treatment, i.e. the patient cannot take an effective deep breath
Nebulized hypertonic saline (3–7%)	● Hypertonic saline nebulizers can be prescribed for use immediately before airway clearance. They can cause bronchoconstriction; thus assess on first use. May not be available out of hours
Inhaled mucolytic drugs, e.g. Pulmozyme	● Cystic fibrosis (CF) patients with tenacious secretions may benefit from inhaled mucolytic drugs, e.g. Pulmozyme. The decision to start using this is not generally made in the on call setting. Mucolytics such as carbocisteine may be considered for all patient groups
Ventilated adult	
Gravity-assisted positioning (GAP)	● GAP with modifications dependent on cardiovascular or neurological impairment
Manual hyperinflation (MHI)	● MHI can be used to augment lung recruitment and mobilize secretions ● An inspiratory hold on the ventilator (if possible) may be useful in those patients unable to tolerate MHI, e.g. PEEP-dependent patients
Suction	● Normal saline is often used to aid clearance of tenacious secretions. Up to 5 ml of 0.9% saline at a time can be instilled via the endotracheal tube or tracheostomy
Humidification	● Humidification is often useful; consider heated systems ● Saline nebulizers can be administered via the ventilator circuit
Manual techniques	● Manual techniques on expiration may assist mobilization of secretions. These can be used in conjunction with MHI or during the expiratory phase of the ventilator cycle

6

Table 6.2 *Continued*

	Suggested treatment options/modifications
Child	● As adults
ACBT	● From 2–3 years upwards with blowing games. Progress to huffing by 3–4 years
Other treatments	● Manual techniques and/or GAP in conjunction with TEEs ● Humidification ● PEP or Flutter may be used at home ● IPPB (consider pressure settings carefully before use). Generally IPPB can be used in children over 6 years ● Exercise as tolerated
Ventilated child	
As above – GAP, MHI and suction as appropriate Humidification	● Humidification with or without a heater may prove useful ● Normal saline is often instilled
Bronchoalveolar lavage	● Therapeutic (non-bronchoscopic) lavage could be considered in children, particularly for upper lobe collapse due to sputum plugging. Do not undertake this procedure unless you have been formally trained to use it
Baby	
GAP	● GAP – if children are not yet walking, sitting should be used if the apical segments are affected
Manual techniques	● Clinically, regular position changes and movement appear to be of benefit in mobilizing secretions ● Infants are unable to participate with TEEs, therefore 30 s percussion with rest periods in between is recommended. This avoids potential associated desaturation ● Shaking and vibrations may not be advisable for self-ventilating babies (see Ventilated baby, below)
Suction	● Nasopharyngeal suction if ineffectively coughing
Ventilated baby	
GAP	● GAP as above
Humidification	● Humidification with or without a heater is essential
MHI	● See paediatric section
Suction	● Suction to clear the secretions

Table 6.2 *Continued*

	Suggested treatment options/modifications
Manual techniques	● Manual techniques can be used. Babies reach functional residual capacity (FRC) at end-expiration. With techniques on expiration it is important to avoid causing collapse – MHI to ↑tidal volume may be helpful ● Saline instillation is useful in clearing secretions from naso/endotracheal tubes <3.0 mm

Modifications for the fatigued patient with increased work of breathing

Adult

Breathing control	● Incorporate additional breathing control and frequent recovery periods during treatment
Positioning	● Positioning to ↓the work of breathing and encourage upper chest relaxation, e.g. sitting forward-lean or high side-lying. Aim for comfort where the upper limbs and/or chest are well supported ● Optimize V/Q matching and thus oxygenation using positioning (in spontaneously ventilating adults position the more affected lung up)
IPPB	● IPPB (high flow rates may be required with very SOB patients) ● Reassurance is essential
Oxygen	● Appropriate oxygen therapy should be discussed with medical staff ● Without altering FiO_2 changes in oxygen delivery method may relieve SOB, e.g. face mask for mouth-breathing patients. Venturi system masks allow delivery of high-flow air and oxygen mixtures even for a relatively low FiO_2. The aim is to provide a higher gas flow rate than the patient's inspiratory requirement
Positive pressure	● IPPB or NIV can reduce WOB and rest the patient. ACBT can be modified for use with NIV in situ. The inspiratory pressure or time can be increased slightly on the ventilator for TEEs, similar to when using IPPB ● NIV may help the patient to tolerate longer treatments and more effective positioning ● CPAP can reduce WOB. It should be used with care if patients are very fatigued and/or at risk of retaining CO_2 (discuss with the medical team). Secretions can become more tenacious. Patients may also have difficulty removing the mask to expectorate. Regular disconnection is detrimental to the benefits gained with CPAP

Table 6.2 *Continued*

	Modifications for the fatigued patient with increased work of breathing
Other issues	● The importance of rest and sleep should not be underestimated ● The sensation of breathlessness can be eased with a fan or open window
Child	● As above
Positioning	● Positioning, V/Q distribution is different in children, see paediatric section
Positive pressure	● NIV incorporating PEEP may be particularly useful as it improves FRC ● CPAP ● IPPB for fatigued children over 6 years
Baby	
Positioning	● Positioning to optimize V/Q and reduce WOB
CPAP	● CPAP is often useful when a baby shows signs of respiratory distress

INEFFECTIVE COUGH (Table 6.3)

Patients with a weak cough find airway clearance difficult and tiring, e.g. patients with:

● neuromuscular disorders
● weak respiratory muscles following prolonged ventilation
● fatigue.

PAIN (Table 6.4)

Pain control is a priority in order to optimize airway clearance.

UNABLE TO COOPERATE (Table 6.5)

Patients may be unable to participate actively in treatment. Confusion, drowsiness or reduced level of consciousness may affect patients' ability to clear secretions.

DEHYDRATION (Table 6.6)

Dehydration can make secretions thicker and difficult to clear.

Table 6.3 Treatments and suggested modifications for ineffective cough

	Suggested treatment options/modifications
Adult	
Increase tidal volume to increase cough effort	● ACBT modified for the individual. With NIV consider a safe increase in inspiratory pressure for TEEs
GAP	● Some patients tolerate head-down or flat positions well whereas others cannot; modify positioning – the use of IPPB or NIV may allow the patient to tolerate these more comfortably
Manual techniques	● Chest percussion, shaking and vibrations can be helpful; however, there is little written evidence of efficacy ● Fatigued patients may tolerate shaking on alternate breaths more easily
Assisted cough techniques	● Assisted cough techniques can be performed supine, side-lying or sitting, as indicated. The force is applied on expiration in the direction of chest wall movement ● Movement such as rolling or positioning may facilitate clearance of secretions (particularly in high-tone patients, e.g. with cerebral palsy) ● IPPB or NIV can be used in conjunction with any of the above ● Cough assist machine (if available) provides a deep breath, followed by cough assistance using negative pressure. This is most effective if used in conjunction with coughing and manual assist techniques
Suction	● If the patient is sufficiently compromised by secretions. Oropharyngeal suction using a Yankuer sucker can be used if secretions are in the mouth. Alternatively oropharyngeal or nasopharyngeal suction may be required. Artificial airways (nasal or oral) can be helpful. Without an airway, nasopharyngeal suction is made easier and more tolerable by using water-soluble jelly ● The risk/benefit of mini-tracheotomy insertion may be considered; check for local hospital policy. Mini-tracheotomy allows clearance of secretions, where nasopharyngeal suction has been beneficial, but is needed frequently. This should be discussed with the medical team

Table 6.3 *Continued*

	Suggested treatment options/modifications
Effective cough	● Paroxysmal coughing can prevent effective clearance of secretions and lead to fatigue or bronchospasm. Advice regarding control of coughing by modification of positioning and breathing control may be helpful. Some patients find swallowing and nose breathing controls paroxysmal coughing
Ventilated adult	● As above ● Assisted cough techniques
Child	● See above section
ACBT, GAP, manual techniques	● ACBT, GAP and manual techniques (see above)
Assisted cough techniques	● Where children have a respiratory rate >40 coordination with expiration can be difficult. Closing volumes are high in children and inspiratory assistance (NIV or IPPB) could be helpful ● IPPB can be considered in children over 6 ● NIV, particularly machines incorporating PEEP, can improve tidal volumes ● Cough assist machine (if available) can be used in children with neuromuscular disease. NB: precautions and contraindications ● High-tone children may benefit from techniques to reduce tone
Ventilated child	● As Table 6.2
Baby	
GAP	● GAP
Manual techniques	● Intermittent chest percussion. It is important to consider closing volume in small children
Suction	● Nasopharyngeal suction may be required; if possible avoid repeated oropharyngeal suction
Ventilated baby	● See Table 6.2

Table 6.4 Treatments and suggested modifications for pain

	Suggested treatment options and modifications
Adult	
Pain control	● Following assessment liaise with medical staff to ensure optimal management of the underlying cause, e.g.:
	a. wound/trauma pain
	b. angina management
	c. management of a pneumothorax
	● Without adequate pain control secretion clearance becomes very difficult. Liaise with medical staff to ensure optimal analgesia. Consider less common analgesics such as Entonox with rib fractures. This must be perscribed and administered by a trained operator
	● Time physiotherapy intervention with the maximal effect of patient's analgesics
	● Modify positioning for comfort
	● Teach postoperative patients wound support techniques for coughing and movement
	● Reassurance and clear explanations regarding treatment and pain control are essential
	● CPAP, e.g. with rib fractures, may help to alleviate pain by splinting the chest wall
	● IPPB appears to be useful when muscular chest wall pain limits TEEs as it makes inspiration a more passive process
Ventilated patient	● Pain may be difficult to assess in sedated patients. Liaise with nursing and medical staff
Child	● See above
	● Liaise with nursing and medical staff to ensure optimal assessment and pain control
Ventilated child	● See above
Baby	● See above
	● The clinical features of pain can be difficult to observe in babies. Appropriate pain scales are available. Liaise with the nursing and medical staff to ensure effective pain relief
Ventilated baby	● See above

Table 6.5 Treatments and suggested modifications for patients unable to cooperate

Suggested treatment options and modifications	
Adult	
Liaise with medical staff to treat the cause of confusion where possible	● A safe level of oxygen therapy to minimize hypoxaemia (SpO_2) ● NIV or ventilation to control hypercapnia ($\downarrow CO_2$) ● Drowsy postoperatively – drugs such as naloxone are sometimes given to reverse the sedative effects of some analgesia. This will also reduce pain control – ensure alternative medication is prescribed ● Confused or disoriented patients need clear and concise explanations. Reassurance during treatment may alleviate anxiety. Minimize distractions, and use appropriate visual prompts
IPPB	● IPPB (where voluntary deep breaths are not achievable). Use a face mask with IPPB if an airtight seal cannot be achieved using a mouthpiece
Manual techniques	● Shaking or vibrations with or without IPPB may be beneficial. Some clinicians advocate chest percussion ● Rib springing or chest compressions can facilitate greater inspiration in unconscious patients ● Neurophysiological facilitation of respiration can be useful in drowsy or unconscious patients. These techniques may increase expansion, alter respiratory rate or facilitate an involuntary cough
Cough assist	● Suction (see Table 6.3)
Ventilated adult	● Clear explanations are required before and during treatment ● Sedation may be necessary to treat fully ventilated patients who are agitated or distressed. Liaise with the intensive care team
Child	● See above ● It is essential fully to involve carers, whose input is often extremely useful ● Some 'unwilling' children can be treated more effectively if distracted or entertained
Ventilated child	● See above
Baby	● Not applicable as babies rarely cooperate!

Table 6.6 Treatments and suggested modifications for dehydrated patients

Suggested treatment options and modifications	
Adult	
Hydration	● Systemic hydration is the priority. Encourage patients to maintain sufficient oral intake. If patients are unable discuss the need for intravenous fluids with medical staff
Humidification	● Use cold water humidification systems with wide-bore tubing to humidify supplemental oxygen. Bubble-through humidification with narrow tubing is not thought to have any objective effect although some patients report a subjective effect ● Heated water humidification systems can be used with self-ventilating patients or those on CPAP or NIV ● Nebulized 0.9% or 'normal' saline solution may be helpful. Sterile water can also be considered but may cause bronchoconstriction ● Ultrasonic nebulizers (with or without heating) can be useful with tenacious secretions (the availability/use of this modality will depend upon local policy)
Ventilated adult	● Systemic hydration is the main priority. Heated water humidification systems can be incorporated into the ventilator circuit ● Saline nebulizers can be administered via the ventilator circuit prior to treatment
Child	● See above – however, ultrasonic nebulizers may not be suitable for children aged less than 6 years
Baby	● Systemic hydration is essential in babies due the high insensible losses ● Head boxes with humidified gas ● Saline nebulizers
Ventilated baby	● See above

BRONCHOSPASM (Table 6.7)

Table 6.7 Treatments and suggested modifications for bronchospasm

Suggested treatment options and modifications	
Adult	
Management of bronchospasm	● Optimal medical management is essential. Well-controlled bronchospasm may allow the patient to clear secretions independently. Medical measures may include inhaled, nebulized or intravenous bronchodilators. Corticosteroids may be required ● Assess inhaler technique where appropriate. A spacer device should be considered ● Time physiotherapy treatment to coincide with the optimal bronchodilator response ● Calm, slow treatments in a comfortable position are essential; avoid repeated coughing and/or huffing as this may worsen bronchospasm ● Manual techniques may increase bronchospasm ● Look out for any signs of fatigue, reducing breath sounds and/or increasing CO_2. Alert medical staff immediately. IPPB or NIV can be very effective in offering some rest; however, this must be discussed with the team to ensure that the deterioration is noted and ICU informed
Ventilated adult	● Instillation of saline could aggravate bronchospasm. Slow instillation is required ● Nebulized bronchodilators can be administered before physiotherapy ● MHI (if used) should stop if bronchospasm increases
Child	● See above section ● IPPB is generally an option for children aged 6 years or more
Ventilated child	● See above section
Baby	● Liaise with medical staff to ensure optimal control of bronchospasm ● Time physiotherapy to coincide with optimal bronchodilator response ● The clinical efficacy of $beta_2$ agonists (i.e. salbutamol and terbutaline) is uncertain in children under 18 months
Ventilated baby	● See above section

Key messages

- The key to effective management is thorough assessment.
- Identify causes of sputum retention not amenable to physiotherapy and liaise with other appropriate members of staff.
- Identify the underlying cause for sputum retention. Treatments selected depend on the individual. Determine which techniques are most appropriate (and you are most confident with) and which are contraindicated.
- Be flexible in your approach to treatment, adapting techniques for the individual. Careful re-evaluation will identify any modifications required.
- Selection of simple outcome measures is essential in evaluating treatment, e.g. SpO_2, respiratory rate, auscultation and volume of secretions.
- Physiotherapy has an important role in the management of sputum retention. Our input in one situation may be advice; in another, intensive treatment.

CHAPTER 7

The management of volume loss

Bernadette Henderson and Nell Clotworthy

There are many diseases and conditions that reduce lung volume; management of these will be covered in this chapter. An accurate assessment will correctly identify which volumes are affected and why. Treatment should be directed at the cause. Remember that not all lung volume loss is amenable to physiotherapy management.

LUNG VOLUMES (Fig. 7.1)

Lung volumes relevant to the on call physiotherapist include functional residual capacity (FRC), tidal volume (V_T) and forced vital capacity (FVC).

FUNCTIONAL RESIDUAL CAPACITY

FRC is the volume of air left in the lungs at the end of a normal expiration. It is the combination of residual volume (RV) and the expiratory reserve volume. RV is the amount of air that cannot be expelled from the lungs at the end of a forced expiration. A 70-kg man would have FRC of approximately 2.4 litres. FRC is influnced by the relationship between the elastic inward recoil of the lungs and the elastic outward recoil of the chest wall.

Causes of decreased FRC

FRC decreases when there is an alteration in the elastic recoil relationship between the lungs and the chest wall. Either there is an:

- increased elastic inward recoil of the lung, e.g. basal atelectasis, fibrosing alveolitis
- loss of elastic outward recoil of chest, e.g. kyphoscoliosis, obesity
- or both.

Reduced FRC can be the result of widespread volume loss, e.g. following abdominal surgery, or more localized loss, e.g lobar collapse. As FRC decreases towards residual volume a point is reached where dependent airways begin to close (closing volume) and remain closed during normal tidal breathing (Fig. 7.2). Gas becomes trapped distal to the closed part of the airway and is rapidly absorbed.

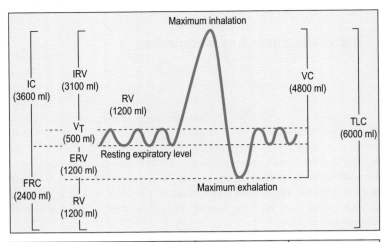

Figure 7.1 Lung volumes. Reproduced with kind permission from Berne and Levy (2000).

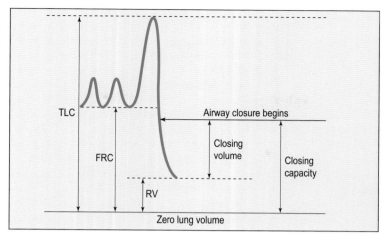

Figure 7.2 Closing volumes. Reproduced with kind permission from Nunn JF (1999) Nunn's applied respiratory physiology. Oxford: Butterworth-Heinemann.

In partial collapse there may be obstruction of airways at normal lung volume, e.g. sputum retention. This results in airway closure and absorption of gas in the lung distal to the obstruction.

Consequences of decreased FRC

Loss of FRC leads to:

● **Reduced lung compliance**.
   a. At normal FRC the lungs operate on the steep part of the pressure/volume (compliance) curve – therefore small changes in distending pressure (by the inspiratory muscles) easily produce an increase in volume (Fig. 7.3A).
   b. At low FRC, lung compliance is reduced (Fig. 7.3B). Tidal volume is less for the same amount of distending pressure. To produce the same tidal volume at low FRC greater inspiratory muscle effort is required – i.e. breathing is harder work. Collapsed lung needs large distending pressures to reinflate it.

● **Altered length–tension relationship in the respiratory muscles.** Muscle has an optimal length for force generation. For a given level of neural stimulation a muscle produces its maximal force at its resting length. If the muscle length increases or decreases there will be a reduction in the force achieved. At normal FRC the inspiratory muscles are at their optimal length. With reduced FRC the diaphragm length increases causing a reduction in force generation.

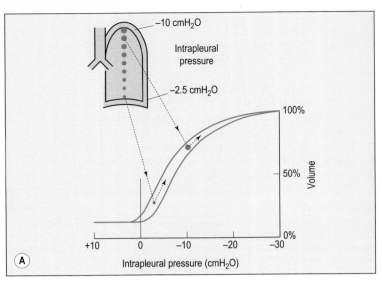

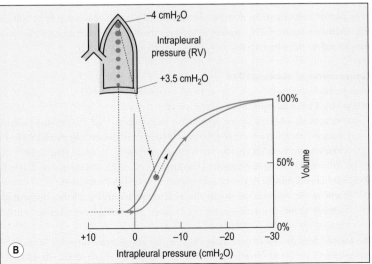

Figure 7.3 Compliance at (A) normal and (B) low lung volume. Reproduced with kind permission from West (2004).

● **Increased airway resistance.** At low lung volumes all air-containing compartments, including the airways, reduce in size. Thus airway resistance increases as lung volume decreases.

> **Remember**
> FRC is important to preserve the surface area for:
> ● gas exchange
> ● V/Q matching
> and therefore oxygenation.

TIDAL VOLUME

Tidal volume (V_T), a normal adult breath, is approximately 500 ml. Tidal breathing starts and finishes at FRC (see Fig. 7.1).

Causes of decreased V_T
● An increase in airway resistance, e.g. bronchospasm, bronchial inflammation
● A decrease in lung compliance, e.g. pleural effusion, fibrosing alveolitis
● A decrease in chest wall compliance, e.g. neuromuscular disorders, pain
● Depression of respiratory drive, e.g. excessive narcotic analgesia.

Consequences of decreased V_T
a. reduction in alveolar ventilation (hypoventilation)
   [Alveolar ventilation = V_T (less dead space) × respiratory rate]
b. carbon dioxide retention and respiratory acidosis
c. hypoxia, if alveolar ventilation is reduced and/or metabolic needs of the body are increased.

FORCED VITAL CAPACITY

FVC is the amount of air that can be forcefully expelled from maximal inspiration to maximal expiration (see Fig. 7.1).

Causes of decreased FVC
● Compromised inspiratory capacity, e.g. reduced inspiratory muscle strength, obesity
● Compromised expiratory capacity, e.g. reduced expiratory muscle strength, increased airways resistance
● Depression of respiratory drive, e.g. neurological impairment.

Consequences of decreased FVC
● Decreased forced expiratory flow rate leading to less effective forced expiration manoeuvres

---

Remember

V_T and FVC are important for:
● CO_2 clearance
● oxygenation
● the ability to huff or cough effectively.

ASSESSING VOLUME LOSS

Consider these questions:
● Which lung volumes are affected (FRC, V_T, FVC)
● Is it generalized or localized?
● Is it:
    a. acute
    b. chronic
    c. acute on chronic loss?
● Which pathophysiological mechanisms are responsible?

Why has the patient got volume loss?

Understanding the underlying pathophysiological mechanisms guides appropriate management (Table 7.1).

Working out the problem

The signs of the different types of volume loss may mimic each other making it difficult to identify the underlying cause.

Table 7.2 lists each of the possible causes together with key assessment 'clues' which should enable the clinician to formulate a working clinical diagnosis. The table also includes a suitable assessment tool for evaluation of treatment success.

Key point of treatment

Once the clinical diagnosis has been correctly established then the following principles of treatment could apply (Boxes 7.1, 7.2, 7.3).

VOLUME LOSS – MANAGEMENT BY DIAGNOSIS

See Table 7.3.

Table 7.1 Underlying pathophysiological mechanisms of volume loss

↓Lung volume due to	Which primary volume affected	Cause
Intrusion of abdominal contents into chest	↓FRC	Position, intestinal obstruction, ascites, paralytic ileus, obesity, congenital defect of the diaphragm, diaphragm paralysis
Abnormalities of the pleural space	↓FRC	Pneumothorax, pleural effusion, empyema, haemothorax
Decrease in chest wall compliance	↓V$_T$, FVC, FRC	**Skeletal problems:** a. kyphoscoliosis b. ankylosing spondylitis **Neuromuscular problems:** fatigue due to increased WOB (length–tension inappropriateness); dystrophies; motor neurone disease; myopathies; spinal injuries; cardiovascular accident (stroke)
Airway obstruction	↓FVC	Secretions, inflammation, collapse, tumour, oedema, bronchoconstriction, foreign body (**NB: paediatrics** – foreign body may cause increase lung volume, i.e. ball valve effect)
Abnormality of lung tissue	↓FRC	Pneumonia, consolidation, upper abdominal and cardiothoracic surgery, interstitial lung disease, collapse, ARDS
Loss of respiratory drive	↓V$_T$, FVC	Neurological impairment, excessive narcotic analgesia
Other factors	↓V$_T$, FVC	Pain (incisional/pleuritic, fractures), fear

Remember

- Do not apply CPAP if the patient is retaining CO_2 – CPAP does not alter V_T and may cause further CO_2 retention and the patient will become more acidotic.
- Consider NIV if the patient is in Type I respiratory failure with a low CO_2 – this may indicate that the patient is working excessively hard, prior to type II respiratory failure.
- Positioning a patient with profound volume loss for treatment may cause desaturation (due to V/Q mismatch) – discuss with the medical team the risk/benefit of increased oxygen therapy while in the position; avoid positions that compromise oxygen saturations if supplementary oxygen is not appropriate.

Table 7.2 Signs and symptoms of volume loss

Condition	History	Chest wall movement	CXR	Arterial blood gases	Auscultation	RR	Lung volume affected	Assessment tool
ARDS/ALI	Many predisposing factors	? reduced	Widespread alveolar shadowing	$\downarrow PaO_2$ $\downarrow SpO_2$?$\uparrow PaCO_2$	Fine inspiratory crackles	$\uparrow$	FRC	PaO_2 SpO_2
Consolidation/ pneumonia	Surgery Infection Immobility Aspiration	? $\downarrow$over area	$\uparrow$opacity (whiter) air bronchograms Loss of silhouette sign	$\downarrow PaO_2$ $\downarrow SpO_2$	Bronchial breathing (BB)	$\uparrow$ or N/A	FRC	PaO_2 SpO_2 Percussion note
Collapse Generalized dependent atelectasis	Surgery Obesity Prolonged recumbency	? $\downarrow$	Raised hemidiaphragms ? opacity in the dependent areas	$\downarrow PaO_2$ $\downarrow SpO_2$	$\downarrow BS$ in dependent areas ? BB	$\uparrow$ or N/A	FRC	Auscultation CXR PaO_2 SpO_2
Collapse	Pain	? $\downarrow$	$\uparrow$opacity	$\downarrow PaO_2$	Absent BS	$\uparrow$	FRC	Auscultation
Lobar	Sputum plugging Incorrect endotracheal tube position	over area	loss of silhouette sign Shift of structures towards opacity	$\downarrow SpO_2$	? BB if patent airway			CXR PaO_2 SpO_2

Flail chest	Chest wall trauma/RTA/fall	Paradoxical	Rib fractures Possible evidence of lung contusion ($\uparrow$opacity)	$\downarrow PaO_2$ $\downarrow SpO_2$	$\downarrow$BS	$\leftarrow$	V_T FVC	PaO_2 SpO_2
Pain	Recent surgery Trauma	$\rightarrow$	Poor inspiratory effort $\downarrow$Lung volume	$\uparrow PaCO_2$? $\downarrow PaO_2$	$\downarrow$BS	$\leftarrow$	V_T FVC	VAS Observation $PaCO_2$
Pleural effusion	Recent surgery Malignancy Heart failure Fluid overload	Normal May be reduced if large effusion	$\uparrow$opacity Meniscal sign Fluid line if erect film (crisp line if air present)	Normal	$\downarrow$BS	$\leftarrow$ if large	FRC	CXR Percussion note
Pneumothorax	Trauma Central line insertion Chest drain removal (occasionally caused by drain being put in to drain an effusion) Idiopathic	$\rightarrow$ Normal	$\uparrow$Translucency (blacker) May be shift of structures away from translucency Increased definition/crispness of heart border or diaphragm indicating anterior and/or basal pneumothorax	$\downarrow PaO_2$ $\downarrow SpO_2$	$\downarrow$BS or absent BS Normal (if small)	$\leftarrow$	FRC ? V_T	CXR RR PaO_2 SpO_2 Percussion note Subcutaneous emphysema

7

Table 7.2 *Continued*

Condition	History	Chest wall movement	CXR	Arterial blood gases	Auscultation	RR	Lung volume affected	Assessment tool
Pulmonary oedema	Evidence of heart failure/renal failure/positive fluid balance	N/A	Widespread alveolar shadowing Bilateral hilar flare ? enlarged heart ? small effusions seen or fluid in fissures visible	↓PaO_2 ↓SpO_2	Late fine inspiratory crackles, wheeze	↑	FRC ? V_T	CXR
Respiratory muscle weakness/ fatigue	Medical diagnosis Extensive period of ↑RR Spirometry – ↓FVC Prolonged ventilatory support	↓ ? Paradoxical if phrenic nerve weakness/ paralysis	Poor inspiratory effort ↓Lung volumes	↑$PaCO_2$? ↓PaO_2 ↓SpO_2	↓BS	↑ or →	? V_T FVC FRC	$PaCO_2$ FVC

7

Box 7.1 Treatment strategies for reduced FRC

Aim: To increase FRC
- Positioning to optimize FRC, V/Q and diaphragm length–tension relationship
- CPAP
- Controlled mobilization with breathing strategies
- If ventilated, increase PEEP

Box 7.2 Treatment strategies for reduced tidal volume

Aim: To increase tidal volume
- Breathing exercises: lower thoracic expansion exercises (LTTEs). Infants cannot significantly increase their tidal volumes so will increase their RR to increase their MV
- Incentive spirometry. In children, blowing games: bubbles/windmills, bubble PEP
- Controlled mobilization with breathing strategies
- IPPB/NIV
- Neurophysiological facilitation techniques
- If ventilated, manual hyperinflation/ventilator hyperinflation when appropriate

Box 7.3 Treatment strategies for localized static volume loss, e.g. lobar collapse

Aim: To reverse atelectasis
- Positioning to optimize FRC, V/Q and diaphragm length–tension relationship
- Advise regarding optimization of O_2 therapy
- Breathing exercises, LTEEs, inspiratory hold, sniff – collateral ventilation, which is not well developed in infants
- Incentive spirometry. In children, blowing games: bubbles/windmills, bubble PEP
- IPPB
- CPAP if good tidal volume
- Controlled mobilization
- Neurophysiological facilitation techniques
- If ventilated, manual hyperinflation
- If secretions present (see Ch. 6)

Table 7.3 Management by diagnosis

Diagnosis	Volume lost	Treatment options	
		Self-ventilating	Ventilated
ARDS/acute lung injury	↓FRC	• Ensure optimization of O_2 therapy • Positioning – erect sitting, side-lying (abdomen free) • CPAP/NIV	• Positioning – side-lying (abdomen free), ?prone • Avoid any manoeuvres which involve disconnecting the patient from the ventilator to preserve PEEP

Consolidation/ pneumonia	↓FRC	• Ensure optimization of controlled O_2 therapy. If severe hypoxaemia may require CPAP or NIV
		• Positioning:
		  Adults – side-lying (abdomen free) with unaffected lung down
		  Paediatrics – side-lying with affected lung down
		  When/if become productive, use airway clearance techniques
		• Humidification
			• Positioning:
			  Adults – side-lying (abdomen free) with unaffected lung down
			  Paediatrics – side-lying with affected lung down
			  When/if become productive, use sputum clearance techniques
			  Paediatrics – may tolerate having the affected lung up which would help drain any loose secretions and encourage ventilation to that lung. As in all patients, need to assess individual's tolerance to handling/treatment

Collapse	↓FRC	• Ensure optimization of controlled O_2 therapy. If severe hypoxaemia may require CPAP or NIV
		• Positioning:
		  Adults – high sitting (bed or chair), side-lying (abdomen free)
		  Paediatrics – as tolerated and manual techniques/ blowing games in younger patients
		• Mobilization with breathing strategies
			• Recruitment manoeuvres – PEEP, manual hyperinflation and inspiratory hold
			• Positioning in high side-lying (abdomen free)
			• Reverse Trendelenburg (feet down, whole bed tilt)
			• Adults – instillation of 0.9% NaCl if sputum plugging
			  Paediatrics – ? selective mini-lavage (if trained) if sputum plugging

Table 7.3 *Continued*

Diagnosis	Volume lost	Treatment options	
		Self-ventilating	**Ventilated**

Collapse lobar	↓FRC	• Ensure optimization of controlled O_2 therapy. If severe hypoxaemia may require CPAP or NIV
		• Positioning:
		  Adults – side-lying (abdomen free) with unaffected lung down (optimize V/Q & GAP)
		  Paediatrics – side-lying with affected lung down (optimize V/Q)
		  May need to have affected lung up to drain. If poorly tolerated short, frequent treatments.
		  Then when improving may tolerate being left with affected lung up to increase ventilation to that lung
		• TEEs with inspiratory holds
		• Neurophysiological facilitation techniques
		• Incentive spirometry (IS)
		• IPPB
		• If sputum retention use airway clearance techniques
			• Positioning:
			  Adults – side-lying (abdomen free) with unaffected lung down (optimize V/Q & GAP)
			  Paediatrics – side-lying with affected lung down (optimize V/Q)
			• Manual hyperinflation maintaining PEEP
			• Inspiratory hold
			• If sputum retention use airway clearance techniques
			  Paediatrics – selective mini-lavage (if trained).
			  If upper lobe problem – sit up provided ETT is well secured

7

Table 7.3 Continued

Diagnosis	Volume lost	Treatment options	
		Self-ventilating	**Ventilated**

Flail chest	$\downarrow V_T$	• Liaise with medical staff to ensure optimal pain control
		• Ensure optimization of controlled O_2 therapy
		• Positioning:
		  Adults – side-lying (abdomen free) with unaffected lung down (optimize V/Q)
		  Paediatrics – side-lying with affected lung down (optimize V/Q)
		• CPAP or NIV to 'splint' the chest wall
		• TEEs with inspiratory holds
		• Neurophysiological facilitation techniques
		• IPPB – avoid use until pneumothorax excluded
		• If sputum retention use airway clearance techniques
			• Positioning:
			  Adults – high sitting or side-lying (abdomen free) with unaffected lung down
			  Paediatrics – high sitting or side-lying with affected lung down but lying on affected side may be more painful and lead to decreased ventilation (unless patient paralysed and fully ventilated with adequate analgesia)
			• If sputum retention use airway clearance techniques

Pain	$\downarrow V_T$
	$\downarrow FVC$
		• Liaise with medical staff to ensure optimal pain control
		• Long acting – e.g. PCA
		  Short acting – bolus of opioid, Entonox
		  Regional analgesia
		• Relaxation techniques
		• Reassurance
			• Lung volumes will not be affected if adequately sedated, analgesed and fully ventilated
			• If on an assisted mode of ventilation, i.e. pressure support & PEEP then:
			  Liaise with medical staff to ensure optimal pain control
			  Long acting – e.g. PCA if awake
			  Short acting – bolus of opioid
			• Relaxation techniques
			• Reassurance

Table 7.3 *Continued*

Diagnosis	Volume lost	Treatment options	
		Self-ventilating	Ventilated

Pleural effusion	↓FVC
	↓V_T if large
		• Positioning:
		  Adults – side-lying (abdomen free) with unaffected lung down (optimize V/Q)
		  Paediatrics – side-lying with affected lung down (optimize V/Q)
		• NB if pleural effusion very large then the above positioning may cause further volume loss – alter to supported high sitting
		• Ensure optimization of controlled O_2 therapy
		• Liaise with medical team regarding insertion of inter-costal chest drain (ICD)
			• Positioning:
			  Adults – side-lying (abdomen free) with unaffected lung down (optimize V/Q)
			  Paediatrics – side-lying with affected lung down (optimize V/Q)
			• Liaise with medical team regarding insertion of ICD

Pneumothorax	↓FVC	• Liaise with medical team regarding insertion of ICD • Ensure optimization of controlled O_2 therapy	• Liaise with medical team regarding insertion of ICD • Ensure optimization of controlled O_2 therapy
Pulmonary oedema	↓FVC	• Ensure optimization of controlled O_2 therapy • CPAP • NIV with CPAP facility • Medical treatment • Positioning in high side-lying (abdomen free) • Reverse Trendelenburg (feet down, whole bed tilt)	• PEEP • Paediatrics – pulmonary oedema may be quite sticky and may potentially cause small airways to block
Respiratory muscle weakness/fatigue	↓FVC ↓V_T	• Fully supported positioning including shoulder girdle • IPPB • NIV	

7

> **Key messages**
> ● Identify which lung volumes are reduced and select the strategy that requires the minimum intervention to produce the required outcome.
> ● Strategies should also include those that can easily be performed independently by the patient or with the help of the nurse.

Further reading

Berne RM, Levy MN (2000) Principles of physiology, 3rd edn. St Louis, MO: Mosby.

Hough A (2001) Physiotherapy in respiratory care: an evidence-based approach to respiratory and cardiac management, 3rd edn. Cheltenham: Nelson Thornes.

Lumb AB (2005) Nunn's applied respiratory physiology. Philadelphia, PA: Elsevier, Butterworth-Heinemann.

Pryor JA, Prasad A (2002) Physiotherapy for respiratory and cardiac problems, 3rd edn. London: Churchill Livingstone.

West J (2004) Respiratory physiology: the essentials. Philadelphia, PA: Lippincott, Williams and Wilkins.

CHAPTER 8

The management of increased work of breathing

Alison Aldridge

This chapter describes the management of patients with increased work of breathing.

> Work of breathing (WOB) = the rate of oxygen consumption of the respiratory muscles

During quiet respiration:
- The work of breathing is performed entirely by the inspiratory muscles.
- Expiration is passive, powered by the elastic recoil of the tissue.
- As breathing becomes more difficult the muscles work harder and thus the WOB increases.

The efficiency of the respiratory muscles is reduced in patients presenting with:
- respiratory disease
- thoracic deformities
- severe obesity, ascites, pregnancy, etc.
- cardiac disease
- cerebral lesions
- sepsis, etc.

Many patients cope with this reduced respiratory muscle efficiency, until something else happens, e.g. chest infection. This results in a much faster deterioration than normal.

CLINICAL SIGNS
See Table 8.1.

BRONCHOSPASM
Bronchospasm is exacerbated by cold, anxiety, dehydration, infection and hypoxia (Table 8.2).

Table 8.1 Clinical features of increased work of breathing

Clinical features of increased work of breathing	

Adult (>16 years)	**Respiratory**
	● ↑RR (dyspnoea)
	● ↓HR (tachycardia)
	● Mouth breathing
	● Altered depth and pattern of breathing (e.g. deep, shallow, irregular, apnoeas, pursed lip breathing)
	● Accessory muscle use
	● Reduced SpO_2
	● Deranged arterial blood gases
	● Carbon dioxide retention (hypercapnia) may cause:
	  a. peripheral vasodilation; warm hands
	  b. bounding pulse
	  c. flapping tremor of hands
	● Secondary signs:
	  a. cerebral – restlessness/irritability/confusion/seizure/coma
	  b. cardiac – tachycardia/hypertension/bradycardia/hypotension/cardiac arrest
	  c. fatigue

Child (>2 years)	**Respiratory** The clinical signs are comparable with those in adults with the following age-related differences: ● ↑RR (tachypnoea) **[2–6 years normal 20–40] [>6 years normal 15–30]** ● Intercostal recession ● Nasal flaring ● Expiratory grunting ● Tracheal tug The secondary systemic clinical signs are similar to those in adults with the following age-related cardiac differences: ● ↑HR (tachycardia) **[normal 60–140]** ● ↑BP (hypertension) **[normal 95–105/53–66]**
Baby (newborn–2 years)	**Respiratory** Clinical signs are comparable to those of a child with the following age-related differences: ● ↑RR (tachypnoea) **[newborn normal 30–50 b.p.m.] [<2 years normal 20–40 b.p.m.]** ● ↑HR (tachycardia) **[newborn normal 80–200 b.p.m.] [<3 years normal 100–190 b.p.m.]** ● ↑BP (hypertension) **[newborn normal 50–70/25–45] [<2 years normal 87–105/53–66]**

8

Table 8.2 Treatments and suggested modifications for bronchospasm

	Suggested treatment options and modifications

Adult	● Check effective bronchodilator therapy, e.g.:
	  a. check technique, regular administration and compliance
	  b. nebulizer therapy requires an adequate tidal volume for effective delivery to the airways – the breathless patient may not receive a therapeutic dose due to small breath size
	  c. intravenous delivery may be more effective (however, potential cardiac side-effects)
	● Use breathlessness positioning to aid relaxation, e.g. forward-lean sitting
	● Ensure adequate, controlled oxygen therapy
	● Humidified oxygen therapy should be prescribed
	● Heated humidification if cold system fails to alleviate bronchospasm
	● Ensure any retained secretions are cleared effectively
	● Active cycle of breathing techniques (ACBT). Emphasis upon breathing control, care with FET as the irritability of the airways may lead to spasms of coughing
	● Avoid manual techniques; single-handed, slow rhythmical percussion can be useful, although evidence is lacking
	● Intermittent positive pressure breathing (IPPB):
	  a. the system should be set up according to local hospital policy and you should only set up and use this equipment if you have been specifically trained and assessed as competent to do so
	  b. bronchodilators can be used in the nebulizer
	  c. use with high flow rate for patient comfort
	  d. try to get patient to rest and let the machine do the work once the breath is triggered
	Note: Discontinue immediately if bronchospasm worsens
	
	● Non-invasive ventilation (NIV):
	  a. the system should be set up according to local hospital policy and you should only set up and use this equipment if you have been specifically trained and assessed as competent to do so
	  b. make sure patient comfortable and reassured
	  c. let patient hold mask to face before being strapped in so that they feel in control
	  d. encourage patient to relax and let the machine help them
	  e. you are aiming to rest the respiratory muscles
	  f. stay with the patient while they become accustomed to the machine

8

Table 8.2 *Continued*

	Suggested treatment options and modifications
	Note: Discontinue immediately if bronchospasm worsens ● Continuous positive airway pressure (CPAP): a. the system should be set up according to local hospital policy and you should only set up and use this equipment if you have been specifically trained and assessed as competent to do so b. in severe asthma hyperinflation of the lungs is common c. in an acute exacerbation, hyperinflation increases as does the WOB d. CPAP takes over the effort of maintaining this sustained inspiratory activity and keeps the airways open during expiration, thus allowing greater gas emptying e. commonly only low pressures are required, 5 cmH_2O, and should be prescribed by medical team, as should the required oxygen level f. the system should be set up according to local hospital policy g. a heated humidification system is recommended **Note: The use of positive pressure in the presence of bronchospasm is controversial and can be technically challenging. It should be undertaken only if discussed with senior medical staff and if you are trained and competent to do so.**
Child	● As above ● Unless using a nebulizer, children between 3 and 5 years are recommended to use an inhaler and spacer; those over 10 years may use a metered dose inhaler ● Consider the use of IPPB in the older child (6 years or older)
Baby	● As above ● Bronchodilator therapy. Unless using a nebulizer, children under 2 years are recommended to use an inhaler with spacer and mask ● Heated humidification is commonly used in the non-intubated baby

8

DISRUPTION OF THE MECHANICS OF THE THORACIC CAGE

See Tables 8.3 and 8.4.

HYPERCAPNIA (PaCO$_2$): TYPE II RESPIRATORY FAILURE

See Table 8.5 and refer also to Chapter 9.

Table 8.3 Disrupted integrity of the thoracic cage

	Suggested treatment options and modifications
Adult	<ul><li>Adequate analgesia</li><li>Controlled oxygen therapy</li><li>Adequate humidification</li><li>CPAP to stabilize a flail segment</li></ul>
Child	<ul><li>As above, although compliance with CPAP is likely to be poor in younger children</li><li>Phrenic nerve damage is a recognized complication post paediatric cardiac surgery resulting in elevation of the diaphragm on the affected side, compression of the lower lobe and persistent collapse</li><li>Physiotherapy is directed towards the management of sputum retention and postoperative atelectasis</li></ul>
Baby	<ul><li>As above; however, in infants prolonged ventilation may be necessary and physiotherapy is directed to managing the presenting problems</li></ul>

Table 8.4 Respiratory muscle weakness

Adult	<ul><li>Phrenic nerve damage is a recognized complication post cardiac surgery resulting in elevation of the diaphragm on the affected side, compression of the lower lobe and persistent collapse</li><li>Neuromuscular weakness affecting the respiratory muscles will gradually present as type II respiratory failure (CO$_2$) due to increasing hypoventilation</li><li>Inadequate nutrition especially in the presence of a prolonged high metabolic rate (e.g. HIV, cancer) decreases the ability to sustain increased respiratory effort – early ventilatory support is beneficial</li></ul>
Child	<ul><li>As above</li></ul>
Baby	<ul><li>As above</li></ul>

Table 8.5 Treatments and suggested modifications for type II respiratory failure

	Suggested treatment options and modifications

Adult	● Hypercapnia PaCO$_2$ >6.0 kPa
	● Consider treatment options for:
	  a. eliminating the identified cause of the hypoventilation, i.e. sputum retention, bronchospasm, etc.
	  b. managing the cause of the hypoventilation, e.g. thoracic/spinal deformity, muscle weakness, distended abdomen, which leaves the patient unable to compensate for a respiratory problem. Ventilatory support is often needed during the acute illness
	● Monitor CO$_2$ and pH regularly. pH below normal levels must be treated – by managing the cause of hypoventilation. Use arterial blood gases or non-invasive transcutaneous CO$_2$ gas monitoring (if available)
	● IPPB. The positive effects of IPPB sessions should be carried over with regular ACBT if possible. You may need to treat the patient little and often. Excellent results are possible with IPPB if NIV is not available to you
	● NIV is an effective treatment to increase CO$_2$ washout, by increasing tidal volume, if available; this must be discussed with the medical team

Child	● As above, hypercapnia PaCO$_2$ >6.0 kPa ● Early detection of mild hypercapnia can be managed by either IPPB or NIV ● The choice of machine and ventilatory setting should be discussed and agreed with the medical team ● Close monitoring of CO$_2$ is essential ● Severe, acute deterioration will require urgent transfer to the paediatric intensive care unit ● Treatment planning will then be directed at eliminating the identified cause of the hypoventilation, i.e. sputum retention, bronchospasm, etc.
Baby	● Hypercapnia PaCO$_2$ >5.0 kPa ● While some NIV machines are suitable for babies, hypercapnia in the very young requires urgent transfer to the paediatric intensive care unit ● Treatment planning is comparable to that for a child, as above

HYPOXIA (LOW O$_2$): TYPE I RESPIRATORY FAILURE

See Table 8.6 and refer also to Chapter 9.

VOLUME LOSS (STATIC AND DYNAMIC)

See Table 8.7.

POSTOPERATIVE RESPIRATORY DYSFUNCTION

The treatment options assume the patient is self-ventilating. Refer to the appropriate chapters for intubated patients (Table 8.8).

Table 8.6 Treatments and suggested modifications for type I respiratory failure

	Suggested treatment options and modifications
Adult	<ul><li>Treat the cause of the low O_2 (hypoxia)</li><li>Continuous saturation monitoring and arterial blood gases as indicated. Saturation monitoring requires good peripheral circulation. Be aware that accuracy is limited by movement, ambient light, nail varnish, as well as underlying pathologies, e.g. anaemias, jaundice, poor peripheral circulation, etc.</li><li>Controlled oxygen therapy to maintain $SpO_2 > 90\%$ (**Check against current BTS guidance**)</li><li>Humidification</li><li>Positioning to maximize V/Q</li><li>If PaO_2 remains around 8 kPa despite FiO_2 0.6 (60%), discuss with medical team. Depending upon assessment findings, consider: a. 100% oxygen, rebreathe bag (remember to close valve to fill bag before use) b. IPPB to increase tidal volume (V_T), or c. CPAP to maximize functional residual capacity (FRC) and oxygenation d. these patients may need to be in a high-dependency environment e. ensure oxygen is available once CPAP/IPPB is removed</li></ul>
Child	<ul><li>Continuous saturation monitoring and arterial blood gases as indicated. The medical team must be made aware of any change in condition</li><li>Controlled oxygen therapy to maintain SpO_2 at 93–98%</li><li>Nasal cannulae are rarely tolerated in young children</li><li>If PaO_2 remains 8 kPa despite FiO_2 0.5 (50%), consider CPAP; however, careful consideration must be given to mechanical support depending on the underlying cause and tolerance of the child</li></ul>
Baby	<ul><li>Monitor as above</li><li>Controlled oxygen therapy. In very young babies it is preferable to maintain the FiO_2 0.6 to minimize risks of oxygen toxicity; discontinue therapy as soon as possible</li><li>Possible methods of delivery are canopy tent, head box, incubator or mask</li><li>Heated humidification is essential</li></ul>

Table 8.7 Treatments and suggested modifications for volume loss

	Suggested treatment options and modifications
Adult	<ul><li>See chapter on volume loss</li><li>Appropriate positioning is essential</li><li>Treatment should be directed at the primary cause</li></ul>
Child	<ul><li>As above</li></ul>
Baby	<ul><li>As above</li></ul>

Table 8.8 Treatments and suggested modifications for postoperative respiratory dysfunction

	Suggested treatment options and modifications
Adult	• Adequate analgesia • Positioning to improve functional residual capacity and distribution of ventilation • Early ambulation • Thoracic expansion exercises with emphasis on 3-second 'hold' and inspiratory 'sniff' to increase tidal volume and collateral ventilation • Incentive spirometry • IPPB if tidal volume still reduced despite above therapies • CPAP if PaO_2 and FRC still reduced despite above therapies
Child	• As above, although care with IPPB and CPAP as compliance may be extremely poor
Baby	• Adequate analgesia. Encourage positioning through play and normal developmental activities, rolling, prone position, etc. • Blowing games in the older baby to facilitate sputum clearance • Severe dysfunction will require prolonged ventilation and physiotherapy is directed to managing the presenting problems

Table 8.9 Treatments and suggested modifications for pulmonary oedema

	Suggested treatment options and modifications
Adult	• Controlled oxygen therapy • Positioning • CPAP. Discuss with the medical team the level of PEEP and FiO_2 to be prescribed • Severe sudden onset of pulmonary oedema will require full ventilatory support and is a medical emergency
Child	• Management depends on severity of the pulmonary oedema • In older children with mild oedema the adult options may be considered. However, if the intrapulmonary shunt is large the child, whatever age, will require urgent transfer to intensive care for mechanical ventilatory support
Baby	Usually a medical emergency due to the large intrapulmonary shunt generated

PULMONARY OEDEMA

Although the pathophysiological cause is not remediable to physiotherapy the consequent hypoxaemia, dyspnoea, tachypnoea and anxiety may respond to intervention while the pharmacological management takes effect (Table 8.9).

SPUTUM RETENTION

Refer to Chapter 6 for the management of sputum retention.

In relation to an acute exacerbation of COPD where sputum retention is the primary cause of an increased WOB, there is evidence to support the short-term use of oral mucolytics (erdosteine or carbocisteine) in the early resolution of symptoms. Whilst this may not be an immediate on call issue it may be raised during the post on call handover for further consideration by the medical team.

Key messages

- Physiotherapy has a pivotal role in the management of increased work of breathing.
- In order to problem-solve and apply clinical reasoning to treatment planning it is easiest to consider that ventilation is the result of a series of interactions between the central control mechanisms, the respiratory muscles, the skeletal structures they influence and the lung tissue itself.
- An increase in the work of breathing may be caused by dysfunction at any one level but it cannot be analysed in isolation, as respiratory mechanics are dynamic in nature.
- Physiotherapy intervention may be directed at more than one point of the system, as dysfunction at one level may disturb, or be compensated for at, other levels.
- The skill is to analyse the major cause of the disruption, based on the presenting clinical features and the results of any relevant clinical investigations, and then decide at which level the chosen treatment will be most effective.

Further reading

Hough A (2001) Physiotherapy in respiratory care: a problem solving approach to respiratory and cardiac management, 3rd edn. Cheltenham: Stanley Thornes.

Prasad SA, Hussey J (1995) Paediatric respiratory care: a guide for physiotherapists and health professionals. London: Chapman & Hall.

Pryor JA, Prasad SA (eds) (2002) Physiotherapy for respiratory and cardiac problems, 3rd edn. London: Churchill Livingstone.

CHAPTER 9

Management of respiratory failure

Sarah Keilty

Respiratory failure is demonstrated in arterial blood gas (ABG) tensions. Type I respiratory failure is defined by a PaO_2 <8.0 kPa with a normal or lowered $PaCO_2$. Type II respiratory failure (ventilatory failure) is defined by a PaO_2 <8.0 kPa and a $PaCO_2$ >6.0 kPa. Acute respiratory failure is related to respiratory distress, with increased work of breathing and deranged gas exchange. It may occur with or without the presence of excessive pulmonary secretions and/or sputum retention, and is not necessarily related to a primary respiratory problem, e.g. neurological problems may be related to respiratory depression, hypoventilation, reduced level of conciousness and inability to protect the airway. Cough depression and risk of aspiration are a serious concern. Unrecognized respiratory failure leads to:

- respiratory muscle fatigue
- hypoventilation
- sputum retention
- $\downarrow O_2$ (hypoxaemia).

Accurate assessment to establish the underlying cause is imperative as, if left untreated, it may progress to any or all of the following:

- cardiac arrhythmia
- cerebral hypoxaemia
- respiratory acidosis
- CO_2 narcosis
- coma
- cardiorespiratory arrest.

Thus timely recognition and treatment of acute respiratory failure is of the utmost importance and a serious part of patient care on call.

HYPOXAEMIA (TYPE I RESPIRATORY FAILURE)

Hypoxaemia is defined as inability to maintain the PaO_2 above 8 kPa. See Box 9.1 and Table 9.1.

Box 9.1 Types of respiratory failure

Respiratory failure is classified in two categories:
- **Type I respiratory failure:** characterized by the inability to maintain an adequate PaO_2 (hypoxaemia) but the $PaCO_2$ is normal (or slightly reduced)
- **Type II respiratory failure** (ventilatory failure): characterized by a reduced PaO_2 and, in addition, the $PaCO_2$ has risen above normal levels (hypercapnia)

Table 9.1 Classification and causes of hypoxaemia

Classification	Cause
Hypoxic hypoxaemia	
• Where blood flows through parts of the lung which are unventilated • Inability to transfer oxygen across the pulmonary membrane (gas diffusion limitation) • Acute bronchoconstriction: asthma (insufficient gas flow in and out of the lung) • Insufficient inspired oxygen therapy (including faulty oxygen delivery equipment)	• Primary respiratory disease: COPD, pulmonary fibrosis, CF, pneumonia, sputum retention, ↓gas transfer across the thickened (fibrotic/oedematous) respiratory membrane • Primary cardiac disease: heart failure, congestive cardiac failure, pulmonary oedema (causing a diffusion limitation across the respiratory membrane)
Ischaemic hypoxaemia:	
• Usually due to inadequate blood flow through the lung	• Pulmonary embolus • Destruction of the pulmonary vasculature (COPD, pulmonary trauma)
Anaemic hypoxaemia:	
• Reduction in oxygen carrying capacity of the blood	• Shock (significant blood loss with a reduced Hb) • Primary haematological diseases, e.g. sickle cell crisis, anaemia
Toxic hypoxaemia:	
• Difficulty in oxygen utilization – common in patients admitted with inhalation burns/smoke inhalation injury	• E.g. carbon monoxide poisoning, cyanide poisoning

CLINICAL SIGNS OF HYPOXAEMIA

A patient with hypoxaemia will display:

- central cyanosis (blue lips, tongue)
- peripheral shut-down (cool to touch, 'cold and clammy')
- tachypnoea – increased respiratory rate (>20 breaths per minute)
- tachycardia (heart rate >100 bpm)
- low oxygen saturation (<90%)
- confusion or agitation if profound hypoxaemia; may not comply with treatment.

AIM OF PHYSIOTHERAPY IN HYPOXAEMIA

- To identify and treat if appropriate the cause of the hypoxaemia, thus aiming to increase the $PaO_2 > 8.0$ kPa while administering appropriate oxygen therapy.

TREATMENT OF HYPOXIA

The primary treatment for hypoxia is controlled oxygen therapy, plus identification and treatment of the underlying cause. Patients who are unable to maintain SaO_2 >90% on facemask oxygen may require additional respiratory support, either continuous positive airway pressure (CPAP) or intubation and mechanical ventilation. See Table 9.2 for treatment advice in hypoxaemia and Table 9.3 for common issues in hypoxaemia. Patients with unilateral lung disease can be positioned in side-lying, with the unaffected lung down, to try to improve V/Q matching.

Table 9.2 Common treatments for hypoxia

Common treatments	Advice
Controlled oxygen therapy	<ul><li>Oxygen is a drug which should be prescribed for the required percentage and/or flow rate</li><li>Usually 24–60% can be given by an oxygen mask</li><li>2–4 L/min via nasal cannulae; however, a mask is preferable if hypoxic and/or mouth breathing</li><li>Over 60% oxygen with persistently low sats (<90%) use a non-rebreathe mask to administer constant flow of high concentration oxygen</li><li>CPAP is useful with profound hypoxaemia once pneumothorax excluded</li></ul>
Humidification	<ul><li>Consider cold or heated humidification</li><li>Heated is better for tenacious secretions or severe bronchospasm</li></ul>
Treat the cause, e.g. bronchospasm, sputum retention, volume loss	<ul><li>If primary respiratory problem, treat this</li><li>If primary problem is cardiac or renal, discuss with the medical team</li></ul>

Table 9.2 *Continued*

Common treatments	Advice
Increased work of breathing	● Use airway clearance techniques if needed ● Positioning is essential to reduce breathlessness and improve ventilation perfusion matching ● IPPB may be useful (with a high flow rate) to rest the muscles and improve efficacy of other treatments

Table 9.3 Common issues in hypoxia

Common issues	Advice
Bronchopneumonia	● Ensure medication is optimized (oxygen, analgesia, bronchodilators, antibiotics, etc.) ● Positioning to decrease work of breathing ● Airway clearance techniques ● Humidification
Acute lobar pneumonia	● During the unproductive phase advice on positioning may reduce WOB ● CPAP is useful for hypoxaemia ● Sputum clearance is only indicated if the patient becomes productive ● *Pneumocystis jiroveci* (previously *P. carinii*) pneumonia (PCP – common in immunosuppressed patients, e.g. HIV) presents with profound hypoxia. CPAP is effective; however, pneumothorax is common – CXR is essential
Pulmonary embolus	● Physiotherapy is not indicated. CPAP may help with severe hypoxaemia
Pulmonary fibrosis	● Present with profound hypoxaemia. Humidified CPAP is effective ● Ensure sufficient oxygen is available when CPAP removed
Pulmonary oedema	● CPAP is effective in treatment of pulmonary oedema. If hypotensive, check that BP does not drop with increased intrathoracic pressure. NIV (pressure support with EPAP) may be useful in the patient tiring on CPAP
CO_2 retention	● Acute CO_2 retention **is not** a reason to reduce the FiO_2 **unless** patients have evidence of acute-on-chronic CO_2 retention secondary to chronic respiratory disease ● This can be diagnosed by interpretation of recent blood gas results, assessing pH, in relation to $PaCO_2$, standard bicarbonate and base excess. Only this group of patients require judicious oxygen administration (24–28%), which should be prescribed accordingly

Table 9.3 *Continued*

Common issues	Advice
Fatigue	● Hypoxaemic patients may start to fatigue. This is seen by a rising $PaCO_2$ – type II failure. An important clinical sign requiring immediate attention. See below
Chronic chest patients	● Patients with longstanding chest disease may have a regular chest clearance routine, e.g. cystic fibrosis, bronchiectatic patients ● Discuss and mould your treatment plan to fit their existing regimen with current physiotherapy problems
Renal failure	● Patients in renal failure may present with ↑WOB ● ABGs will show metabolic acidosis, generally with some respiratory compensation – i.e. ↓CO_2 (due to high RR) ● Pulmonary oedema and pleural effusion may be present
Distended abdomen, e.g. pancreatitis, ascites	● Positioning in alternate side-lying or well-supported high side-lying is useful ● Standing if possible
Oesophageal varices	● Dilated blood vessels in oesophagus may rupture with increased pressure ● Care with coughing; suction contraindicated ● Prevent chest infection by positioning, teach huff, mobilize if able

HYPERCAPNIA (TYPE II RESPIRATORY FAILURE/VENTILATORY FAILURE)

Acute ventilatory failure can be caused by problems in several systems other than the respiratory system. Retention of carbon dioxide reflects hypoventilation. This is caused by a reduction in the extent and efficiency of gas mixing in alveoli and is primarily caused by inadequate alveolar ventilation. Any pathology affecting tidal volume and respiratory rate will affect gas mixing in the alveoli.

A slight rise in arterial CO_2 will produce a response – increasing ventilation by a rise in either respiratory rate, tidal volume or both. If this response is marked and the respiratory rate is >25/minute the work of breathing is high. The increased muscle work cannot be sustained for long periods and respiratory muscles begin to fatigue. In this case, patients develop a rapid shallow breathing pattern whereby tidal volume is reduced resulting in an inability to move little more than dead space volume (e.g. 150–200 ml). This means that CO_2 cannot be adequately 'washed out' of the lung resulting in CO_2 retention. This causes the following signs and symptoms:

● A surfeit of hydrogen ions producing a respiratory acidosis.

● Agitation and acute confusion.

● Patients may look flushed and peripherally dilated with a 'bounding' pulse (CO_2 is a potent vasodilator).

● Patients may exhibit hand tremor known as CO_2 related 'flap'.

● When CO_2 retention is profound, the patient is drowsy and difficult to rouse and respiratory rate is often reduced (<10 breaths per minute). This is CO_2 narcosis which is a likely cause of CNS depression. NB: If the GCS is equal to or less than 9, the patients may not be able to protect their airway, so anaesthetic advice should be sought. Intubation and invasive mechanical ventilation may be indicated, especially with primary neurological pathology. See Table 9.4 for causes of acute ventilatory failure.

Table 9.4 Causes of acute ventilatory failure

Causes of acute hypoventilation and carbon dioxide retention (acute ventilatory failure)	Explanation
CNS depression	● Opiates used for pain relief, sedation and drug abuse. Check renal function if on small dose and patient appears drowsy. Tell-tale sign is the presence of pinpoint pupils bilaterally ● Alcohol ● Head injury
Respiratory disease	● Fatiguing respiratory muscles due to ↑work of breathing with a rapid shallow pattern ● Poor functioning respiratory membrane ● Oxygen >28% in chronic CO_2 retaining patients
Neuromuscular blockade	● Anaesthesia ● Ingestion of poison
Muscle weakness – inability to sustain increased respiratory loads	● Muscle diseases ● Fatigue ● Long-term steroids ● Metabolic abnormalities (renal, liver impairment)
Loss of integrity/restriction of the chest wall – poor pulmonary mechanics	● Pain ● Circumferential burns to the thorax ● Thoracic trauma ● Thoracic cage deformity (kyphoscoliosis) ● Previous thoracic surgery

Table 9.4 *Continued*

Causes of acute hypoventilation and carbon dioxide retention (acute ventilatory failure)	Explanation
Neurological impairment	● Upper motor neurone lesions (CVA, head injury) may affect respiratory rhythm and pattern ● Lower motor neurone lesions (polio, multiple sclerosis, motor neurone disease, etc.) ● Neuromuscular junction (myasthenia gravis) ● Problems as for muscle weakness (above)

TREATMENT OF HYPERCAPNIA

Treatment of ventilatory failure usually requires respiratory support in order to increase tidal volume and/or respiratory rate (i.e. minute ventilation) (Table 9.5). This can be intubation and ventilation or non-invasive ventilation (NIV) with a face mask. NIV is the treatment of choice for patients with acute ventilatory failure with a GCS > 9–10, provided there is no primary neurological pathology and they can protect their airway. For patients with chronic respiratory disease if the poor

Table 9.5 Common treatments for hypercapnia

Common treatments	Advice
Identify and ensure treatment of the *cause* of the hypoventilation	● If the patient is on an opiate infusion, assess sedation status especially in the elderly or patients with reduced renal/liver function as they will not be able to excrete opiates at a normal rate. In discussion with the medical team opiate infusions should be reduced or stopped, and reversing agents (e.g. naloxone) administered in severe cases. Alternative pain control should be found ● Severe bronchospasm and sputum retention need immediate, careful treatment ● If the cause is untreatable, e.g. Guillain-Barré, ventilation must be considered
The primary treatment for acute, severe CO_2 retention is to increase the minute ventilation, without an increase in the total work of breathing	● If respiratory rate is high this can only be achieved by increasing tidal volume. In order to do this assisted ventilation of some form is needed, e.g. IPPB, NIV ● IPPB will ↓WOB and ↑TV, thereby ↑O_2 and ↓CO_2, increasing efficacy of cough (due to greater TV) during treatment. NIV will offer the same effect continuously ● If sputum retention is the cause, short regular treatment is invaluable, incorporating IPPB, manual techniques, assisted cough and positioning

Table 9.5 *Continued*

Common treatments	Advice

Non-invasive ventilation	● Patients who do not respond to the above strategies may retain CO_2 and become acidotic. Non-invasive ventilation (NIV) should be considered if the resources and training are available; otherwise full ventilation will need to be discussed
	● NIV allows correction of CO_2, acid–base balance by increasing alveolar ventilation. NIV offloads some of the work of the respiratory muscles, allowing a degree of respiratory muscle rest. NIV is a mode of respiratory support rather than a treatment modality and is tolerated for protracted periods
	  a. the system should be set up according to local hospital policy and you should be specifically trained and competent to do so
	  b. check for contraindications
	  c. discuss settings with the medical team
	  d. correct mask fitting is essential for effective NIV:
	    – leave false teeth in situ to maintain normal facial shape and tone
	    – watch for potental leaks, e.g. around NG tubes
	    – prevent tissue breakdown on the bridge of the nose, by ensuring good fit
	    – avoid air blowing into the eyes
	  e. Consider the need for additional humidification to prevent bronchospasm, secretion retention and further exacerbation of hypercapnia
	  f. Entrain supplemental oxygen through the inspiratory limb of the ventilator in preference to a side port on the mask, and measure with an oxygen analyser
	  g. Set the required minimum respiratory rate in case of complete apnoea due to oxygen therapy
	  h. Monitor regularly for mask leaks, discomfort, claustrophobia, skin damage and gastric distension
	  i. Discuss a management plan with the nursing staff, including how often to come off for drinks, cough, pressure area care, etc.
	  j. Ensure repeat gases are taken 20–30 minutes after stabilization to check effect upon the hypercapnia/acidosis. If no effect check with medical team and change settings in line with agreed local policy
	  k. Gradually reduce time spent on treatment as indicated by the clinical condition and as independent ventilation becomes more effective at maintaining gas exchange
	● Full ventilation has the same effect

GCS is as a result of CO_2 narcosis (look for evidence of elevated CO_2 and bicarbonate ions in the blood gas) – then a trial of NIV may be appropriate, provided a plan has been put in place for intubation if there is no improvement in the first 30 minutes and it is carried out in the intensive care unit with early access to intubation. In mild hypercapnia, intermittent positive pressure breathing (IPPB) may be adequate to improve alveolar ventilation in the short term – as this is an intermittent treatment it is unlikely that severe hypercapnia will be reversed. See Table 9.6 for common issues in hypercapnia.

Remember acute ventilatory failure can be caused by problems in several systems other than the respiratory system. However, it is important to stress that it may be caused by an acute deterioration of a chronic condition – it is helpful to read the patient's old notes to establish what the patient's usual status is – see section on chronic ventilatory failure.

Table 9.6 Common issues in hypercapnia

Common issues	Advice
Low pH	● Once pH dips below normal range urgent treatment from the whole team is needed
Call to A&E	● You may be called to resus in A&E as this client group benefit from timely physiotherapy intervention ● Do not be scared by this – treat it as a ward, with more help on hand ● Start your treatment here
No access to IPPB, CPAP, NIV in ward area	● If a patient requires positive pressure for treatment and no other treatment options remain, they must be moved to an appropriate area – the medical team should be able to arrange this ● If your hospital does not have access to CPAP, IPPB or NIV treat the patient to the best of your ability using the techniques available to you. Often excellent results are possible. If the patient needs more assistance ICU support will be required – inform the medical staff as to the limitations of your treatment
High probability of death	● If the team establish that death is the most likely outcome, the need for treatment must be weighed up against the discomfort felt by the patient and their needs, e.g. time with family

CAUSES OF CHRONIC CO$_2$ RETENTION (CHRONIC VENTILATORY FAILURE)

Patients with chronic respiratory disease may have chronic CO$_2$ retention. This is identified from blood gas analysis where the PaCO$_2$ is >6.5 kPa, the pH is normal and the bicarbonate (HCO$_3$) is also elevated above 28 mmol/l. If these patients develop 'acute-on-chronic respiratory/ventilatory failure', they will retain more CO$_2$ but the pH will fall as there will be insufficient time for the kidneys to retain bicarbonate ions to correct the acidosis. NIV is the treatment of choice in this situation, bearing in mind the cautions mentioned above. See Table 9.7 for causes of chronic ventilatory failure and Table 9.8 for common medications.

Table 9.7 Causes of chronic ventilatory failure

Respiratory disease	● Inadequate alveolar ventilation due to fatiguing respiratory muscles; inadequate surface area for gas exchange
Cardiac disease	● Cardiac failure (LVF/CCF) and pulmonary oedema increase respiratory work, with poor oxygenation of the respiratory muscles
Neurological diseases	● Inadequate respiratory muscle strength and endurance
Muscle problems	● As for neurological, above ● Profound malnutrition ● Hyperinflation alongside respiratory disease
Sleep-related breathing disorders	● Severe, longstanding obstructive sleep apnoea, nocturnal hypoventilation/central sleep apnoea

Table 9.8 Common medications

Common medication effects	Examples of medication
Bronchodilators	● Nebulized: salbutamol, terbutaline, ipratropium bromide ● Intravenous: salbutamol, aminophylline
Corticosteroids	● Nebulized: beclometasone ● Oral: prednisolone
Diuretics	● Furosemide (frusemide)
Anticoagulants	● Tinzaparin, heparin
Anti-arrhythmics	● Digoxin, amiodarone, adenosine

Key messages

- Treatment must be aimed at the cause of the hypoxia and/or hypercapnia so that deranged gas exchange can be corrected and work of breathing reduced.
- Respiratory support in the form of oxygen and positive-pressure techniques can support the patient while physiotherapy techniques may expedite recovery.

Further reading

BTS Guideline (2002) Non-invasive ventilation in acute respiratory failure. Thorax 57: 192–221.

Davidson C, Treacher D (eds) (2002) Respiratory critical care, 1st edn. London: Edward Arnold.

West JB (2004) Respiratory physiology: the essentials, 6th edn. London: Lippincott Williams & Wilkins.

West JB (2007) Pulmonary pathophysiology: the essentials, 7th edn. London: Lippincott Williams & Wilkins.

CHAPTER 10

Calls to adult intensive care

Rachel Devlin

The purpose of this chapter is to highlight different terminology, equipment and specific issues pertinent to the intensive care patient. This chapter will cover:

● Considerations in the assessment of the ICU patient
● The environment
● Common pathologies
● Physiotherapy management.

Calls to an intensive care unit (ICU) can be nerve-wracking due to the complexity of the environment, the variety of pathologies encountered and the severity of the patient's condition. However, remember that this is a safe environment for you as all ICU patients are closely monitored. There is a higher proportion of nursing staff to patients, and staff are highly skilled and can offer a wealth of advice and assistance in an on call situation, e.g. explaining unfamiliar terminology.

It is important to remember that critically ill patients may be anywhere in the hospital. As such, critical care should be viewed as a concept, rather than a location. You may be the first person to locate such a patient and in that case you should not be afraid to call for help. Many units have recognized this and have developed 'critical care outreach teams' to support staff. You should check your local policies to see if your unit has an outreach team and how to access them.

SPECIAL CONSIDERATIONS FOR ASSESSING ICU PATIENTS

Remember!
The basic components of respiratory assessment remain the same regardless of whether the patient is on ICU or on a ward. See Chapter 2. Using a logical format allows you to identify whether the patient has (or is at risk of developing) loss of lung volume, sputum retention or increased work of breathing leading to respiratory failure (see also Chapters 6–9).

GENERAL
● What is the patient's global stability and response to handling?
● What has happened since admission/last treatment (e.g. intubation, lines inserted)
● What physiological parameters are the medical team working towards?
● Note the equipment attached to the patient, e.g. drips and drains.
● Are there any limitations to movement or positioning (e.g. due to attachments, equipment or spinal stability – see Chapter 14).

CVS
● What is the patient's heart rate/rhythm? Is it compromising their blood pressure? What effect is your treatment likely to have on this?
● Is BP stable? Are they on any inotropic support?

CNS
● Is the patient sedated? Are they on any paralysing agents?
● What is the patient's level of consciousness? (sedation scoring, AVPU, GCS)
● Is analgesia sufficient for full assessment and treatment?
● Is there any neurological deficit evident? If so, is swallow/cough reflex affected? (see Chapter 14).

BIOCHEMISTRY
● What is Hb?
● Is clotting deranged? (look at platelets/INR/PT/APTT)
● Are there signs of infection/sepsis? (WCC/CRP/lactate)

RENAL
● What is current urine output? Overall fluid balance?
● Is the patient on any renal support? (diuretics, haemofiltration)

RS
● Mode of ventilation and method of delivery?
● Ventilator settings?
● Level of oxygen? Saturations?
● Does the patient have a cough? Sputum on suction? Colour, volume and consistency? Clearing easily with suction?
● Are there chest drains in situ? What are they there for?

A few additional factors need to be considered before you continue:

- Anxiety
  - Explain all interventions to the patient regardless of their sedation level in order to minimize anxiety – there is good evidence that patients can hear what is happening.
- Relatives
  - Friends and relatives will find this environment very stressful. This can manifest itself in many ways. Always remain calm and professional, listen to what they have to say – they can be an advocate for you with the patient. But remember you are there to treat the patient and do what you and the team feel is most appropriate for their care.
  - Make sure you know who you are talking to and respect your patient's confidentiality.
  - Discuss your role with the patient's relatives, but try to avoid having conversations about medical plans, prognosis, etc. This is the role of ICU staff.
- Expectations
  - Patients in ICU are by definition critically ill; therefore there may be a high probability of death. Try to be realistic in your expectations of yourself.
  - Balance the probable benefit of your treatment against the discomfort, time and energy that it may require of the patient.
  - On occasion, when a patient has been weaned from support and extubated, the decision is made that the treatment will not be escalated should their condition deteriorate. In a small number of cases where the patient will not survive their illness, the ET tube may be removed and the patient made comfortable as part of the palliative process.
- The unfamiliar
  - When encountering unfamiliar pathologies with an uncertain prognosis, it is important not to pre-judge the outcome of their ICU stay. Ask the nursing staff what to expect of the underlying pathology and consider any potential contraindications for physiotherapy treatment.

During your induction to on call you should familiarize yourself with the equipment commonly used within ICU. Before approaching the patient, note the equipment, lines, etc. that are attached to the patient and the precautions/care you should take.

Remember!
If you are unsure of any equipment or lines ask for help/explanation from ICU staff.

THE ENVIRONMENT

ICU has many pieces of equipment – Table 10.1 gives a brief summary of some of the common items you will see.

With lots of equipment come lots of different alarm systems. For equipment such as infusion pumps it is vital you do not switch them off. However, it is helpful to nursing staff if you can identify the cause of the alarm. For monitoring and ventilators Table 10.2 highlights some of the common causes of alarms in ICU and how you should manage them. Do not switch off alarms unless you are competent to identify the cause and manage appropriately. If in doubt, ask!

Table 10.1 ICU equipment

Equipment	Explanation
Arterial line – blood pressure monitoring	● Inserted via radial, brachial or dorsalis pedis arteries ● Care with positioning to avoid disconnection or kinking of lines (may make the trace unreliable) ● Liaise with nursing staff regarding reliability of the trace ● Blood pressure cuffs may also be used
ECG electrodes – heart rate and rhythm monitoring	● Take care with techniques that may disrupt the trace and set off the alarms, e.g. manual techniques ● Always remember to check the 'stickies' if the trace changes
CVP (central venous pressure) line – monitors pressure in the right side of the heart	● Commonly inserted in the internal jugular or subclavian vein ● Drugs may be administered via the CVP line; if so the measurement will be inaccurate. Take care not to kink the line during turning as drug delivery may be affected ● Risk of pneumothorax during insertion; therefore ensure that patient has a CXR prior to using positive pressure adjuncts, e.g. IPPB, MHI
Invasive cardiac monitoring/ equipment (e.g. PA catheter, PiCCO/LiDCO, intra-aortic balloon pump (IABP), pacing wires)	● Refer to Chapter 15 ● Check with staff on stability of patient and limitations to movement/positioning ● There are similar risks with the insertion of PA catheters as with CVP lines
Invasive neurological monitoring/ equipment (e.g. ICP bolt, extraventricular drains (EVD) or cerebral function monitors (CFM))	● Refer to Chapter 14 ● Check with staff on stability and limitations to positioning

10

Table 10.1 *Continued*

Equipment	Explanation
Haemofiltration (HF) – renal failure. May also be documented as CVVHF or CVVHD	● Vas-Cath (a large-bore double-lumen cannula) inserted into the subclavian or internal jugular vein (for neck), or femoral veins (for groin) ● Take care not to kink lines – will affect function of machine. Do not flex the hip greater than 30–45° if femoral line ● Check with staff on stability and other limitations to positioning ● There will be changes in overall fluid status with patients on renal support that may predispose them to cardiovascular instability
Airways Endotracheal tube (may be oral or nasal), tracheostomy tube	● Endotracheal tube used initially ● Nasal ETT may suggest a difficult intubation – so take care ● Tracheostomy may be used to wean from mechanical ventilation. See tracheostomy section in Chapter 13 ● Ventilated patients will have a cuffed airway in place. If a patient is able to vocalize or there are audible oral noises, inform the nursing staff as there may be a cuff leak which may affect ventilation
Ventilators Be aware of the different types of ventilator in use in your hospital. It is of note that a variety of ventilatory parameters can be changed in order to optimize gas exchange and minimize the potential damage to the lungs	● Different manufacturers of ventilator have different names for the modes of ventilation (e.g. BiPAP, PRVC, ASB, etc.). Often the full name will give you a clue as to the type of ventilation this is ● Controlled modes of ventilation – the patient makes little or no respiratory effort. This may indicate a more acute or severe condition, e.g. head injury or sepsis ● Supported modes of ventilation allow the patient to trigger the ventilator, namely that they are able to initiate some breaths. This indicates that the patient's condition is improving or less severe. These modes can be used while weaning ventilation (decreasing respiratory support) ● Modern machines will allow a patient to breathe on top of a controlled mode of ventilation. To see if a patient is doing this, look at the set breathing rate and then the actual breathing rate on the ventilator
Non-invasive ventilation/CPAP	● See Chapter 9

10

10

Table 10.2 Common causes of alarms in an ICU and their management

Problem	Potential causes	Physiotherapy management
Reduced lung volumes May alarm as: ● Decreased tidal volume ● Decreased minute volume ● Decreased SpO₂ ● Increased peak airway pressure	● Leak in circuit ● Dislodged ETT ● Excess water in circuit ● Sputum plug ● Acute lung injury	● Check connections in circuit ● Consider repositioning ● Suction or further physiotherapy intervention ● Patient may require increased FiO₂
Increased work of breathing May alarm as: ● Decreased tidal volume ● Decreased minute volume ● Increased respiratory rate	● Bronchospasm ● Patient waking/biting on tube ● Patient waking up and making increased respiratory effort ● Increased respiratory rate, e.g. due to pain, anxiety or fatigue	● Analgesia, reassurance, sedation or increased ventilatory support ● Nebulized bronchodilators
Sputum retention May alarm as: ● Increased peak airway pressure ● Decreased SpO₂ ● Decreased tidal volume	● Sputum plug ● Patient waking up/coughing	● Suction or further physiotherapy intervention ● Patient may require increased FiO₂
Respiratory failure	● Could be any combination of the above	● Needs review of ventilator settings

Monitor alarming

Decreased blood pressure	• Unreliable arterial line trace • Kinked lines • Due to bleeding • Following nursing intervention, e.g. turning • During physiotherapy intervention, e.g. MHI or manual techniques • Due to increase/bolus of sedation	• If unreliable, use blood pressure cuff • Ensure lines are patent for effective delivery of drugs, e.g. inotropes • Patient may require intravenous fluids/surgical opinion • Observe if BP returns to normal. If not, return patient to supine. If low BP persists, patient may require intravenous fluids or inotropes • Stop technique and allow patient to settle; BP should recover quickly. If not, discuss further intervention with nursing staff. One treatment at a time may be possible or there may be a medical solution to support BP during treatment • Administer intravenous fluids or decrease sedation if appropriate
Increased blood pressure	• Pain • Anxiety	• Analgesia • Sedation or reassurance
Increased heart rate	• Infection • Decreased blood volume, e.g. bleeding, haemofiltration • Pain • Anxiety	• Investigation and treatment of underlying cause • Patient requires medical review • Analgesia • Sedation or reassurance

10

10

Table 10.2 *Continued*

Problem	Potential causes	Physiotherapy management
Decreased heart rate	● Due to medication, e.g. beta-blockers, sedatives ● Due to vagal stimulation, e.g. following suction or movement of ETT	● Patient may require medical review ● Monitor response to further interventions and discuss with medical team
Arrhythmias, e.g. atrial fibrillation (ensure nursing staff are aware of any change in ECG trace)	● Hypoxia ● Sepsis	● Patient may require anti-arrhythmic drugs, e.g. amiodarone, or cardioversion to restore sinus rhythm ● Treatment of underlying cause
Decreased SpO$_2$	● Unreliable trace ● Sputum retention ● Decreased lung volume or V/Q mismatch ● Fluid overload	● Check reliability of trace (i.e. HR from pulse oximeter and ECG trace should match). If poor, relocate probe, e.g. to toes, earlobes ● Suction or further physiotherapy intervention ● Consider repositioning or further physiotherapy intervention ● Diuretics, inotropes, renal support ● Patient may require increased FiO$_2$

COMMON PATHOLOGIES/CONDITIONS IN ICU

Table 10.3 summarizes some of the common pathologies and conditions seen within the ICU.

As part of your assessment you will also note that the patient may be receiving a number of drugs with which you are unfamiliar. Common drugs encountered in intensive care are described in Appendix 4. Bringing together all the information that you have gathered from your assessment will help you to identify the patient's individual problem and allow you to develop a treatment plan (Table 10.4).

Table 10.3 Common ICU pathologies and conditions

ARDS (acute respiratory distress syndrome)/ALI (acute lung injury)	● Syndrome characterized by reduction in lung compliance and need for high PEEP and oxygen requirements but as it is an interstitial pathology secretions are not generally a problem ● Caution with hands-on techniques as you do not want to de-recruit lung units (i.e. lose the splinting effect of the ventilator PEEP) ● Treatment may consist of positioning only, e.g. prone-lying to optimize gaseous exchange ● If secretions become a problem ensure adequate humidification along with other techniques to improve sputum clearance
Sepsis – systemic inflammatory response syndrome (SIRS)	● Normal WBC = $4–11 \times 10^9$/L; ↑WBC indicates infection ● CVS instability, e.g. decreased BP, will occur and patient may require cardiac support drugs or fluid management to maintain adequate perfusion ● Positioning or MHI may be contraindicated as these may compromise BP ● Urine output may decrease leading to fluid overload and pulmonary oedema. This will compromise oxygenation and the patient may require high FiO_2 and increased PEEP ● If there are signs of pulmonary infection, try one treatment at a time, e.g. side-lying, and monitor the patient's CVS response
Unilateral lung pathology, e.g. pneumonia	● Self-ventilating patient – See Chapter 12 ● Intubated patients – Remember V/Q. IPPV changes the dynamics of ventilation and air is forced into area of least resistance. Therefore the airways which are open more tend to get overstretched. In a side-lying patient the non-dependent area (upper lung) receives greater ventilation. Perfusion is unchanged in the ventilated patient

10

Table 10.3 *Continued*

	● If the affected lung is dependent, desaturation may occur due to poor perfusion. If it is non-dependent, desaturation may occur because the disease process limits gas exchange secondary to secretions. You need to assess each patient on an individual basis and establish appropriate positions for treatment, which may be different to the position you leave the patient in
Head injuries, neurosurgery and spinal cord injuries	● Refer to local hospital guidance on management ● See Chapter 14
Spinal fractures/ orthopaedic trauma	● See Chapters 13 and 14 ● Long bone fractures may cause fat emboli leading to type I respiratory failure ● **Log rolling only until a full set of spinal films has been performed and the spine cleared; medical staff must document if patient can be positioned in any position other than supine** ● Note orthopaedic instruction for peripheral fractures
Rib fractures/flail segment/sternal fractures/lung contusions	● Be aware of fracture sites ● For management see Chapter 15
Burns	● Ensure that the patient has effective pain relief and adequate humidification as secretions may be thick and difficult to clear ● Early, regular chest clearance is vital to remove soot (etc.) particles from the lungs. Soot around the nose and mouth is suggestive of inhalation injury which results in oedema and sputum ● Patients with large-scale burns will require rapid fluid replacement and so are prone to pulmonary oedema ● **If stridor occurs, seek urgent medical advice due to risk of airway obstruction** ● Postural drainage is contraindicated in the presence of head/neck oedema ● Check local policies with regard to movement and manual techniques over skin grafts. Some units allow this once the graft is established provided that the graft is healthy and there is thick padding over the affected area. Check with the on call team covering the specialty which undertook the surgery

Table 10.3 *Continued*

	• Escharotomy of the chest wall; effective chest care is essential – however, analgesia is vital • Burns patients are immunosuppressed, so it is vital to adhere to infection control policies • Many units require that passive movements to affected areas are continued for burns patients at weekends – check local policy
Clotting disorders	• If INR >1.0 (associated with anticoagulants or liver dysfunction) or in the presence of DIC (disseminated intravascular coagulation), bleeding may occur leading to cardiovascular instability • Secretions may be blood stained and care should be taken if performing suction to minimize trauma. Manual techniques may be contraindicated • If INR <1.0 there will be a predisposition to clotting, e.g. DVT, PE • A falling platelet count may be a sign of sepsis. Low platelets predispose to bleeding and therefore care should be taken during all interventions to minimize trauma to the patient, e.g. when repositioning the patient
Postoperative patients	• Effective pain relief is essential to ensure patient compliance with treatment • Important to observe surgical instructions regarding positive pressure adjuncts, positioning and mobilization • See Chapter 13
Respiratory medical patients	• See Chapter 12 • Aim to prevent patient fatigue by management of increased work of breathing and sputum retention • NIV may be considered. Setting up NIV may not be the role of the on call physiotherapist, so it is important to be aware of hospital policy
Renal failure patients	• See Chapter 12 • A patient may present with respiratory problems, e.g. increased RR, but blood gas analysis shows that it is a compensatory mechanism for a primary metabolic problem, e.g. acute renal failure • Patient may be admitted for haemofiltration; see Chapter 12 • Main problem is commonly pulmonary oedema leading to type I respiratory failure. This may respond to diuretics and CPAP

10

Table 10.4 Management of ICU problems

Problem	Cause	Physiotherapy management	Further management
Sputum retention	Poor cough, pain, dehydration, fatigue	Sputum clearance techniques	Decrease sedation, ensure adequate analgesia, increase respiratory support, e.g ↑pressure support
Bronchospasm	Previous respiratory disease, sputum retention, fluid overload, renal failure, anxiety	Sputum clearance techniques. Positions to relieve breathlessness, reassurance	Bronchodilators, diuretics, haemofiltration
Lobar collapse	Sputum plug, migration of ET tube, position in bed	Sputum clearance techniques. Mobilization, e.g. sitting out	Reintubation, bronchoscopy. Rehydration
Pulmonary oedema	Cardiac or renal failure	*Physiotherapy is NOT indicated for pulmonary oedema*	Inotropic support, e.g. epinephrine; diuretics, e.g. furosemide. Fluid restriction. Haemofiltration
Pulmonary embolus (PE)		*Physiotherapy is NOT indicated for a PE. Do NOT mobilize patient without discussing with doctors*	Anticoagulation, TED stockings
Pleural effusion	Cardiac/renal failure. Fluid overload. Malignancy	*Physiotherapy is NOT indicated for a pleural effusion, although patient may respond to positions to relieve breathlessness if symptomatic*	Diuretics, intercostal chest drain. See Chapter 18
Pneumothorax	Spontaneous, e.g. Marfan syndrome. Traumatic, e.g. stabbing	Encourage mobilization	Analgesia. Intercostal chest drain if symptomatic. See Chapter 18
Fatigue	As described previously	Sputum clearance techniques, positions to decrease breathlessness, reassurance	Treatment of underlying cause. Non-invasive ventilation, intubation and ventilation, increasing respiratory support. Sedation, e.g. propofol

Key messages

- Approach assessment of the ICU patient in the same systematic and logical format that you would use to assess a ward patient.
- Work closely with the nursing and medical staff.
- Communicate the outcome of your assessment and treatment succinctly.
- Don't be afraid to ask questions.
- Don't be scared!

Acknowledgements

The author would like to acknowledge the input of Sara Smailes in the burns section of this chapter.

Further reading

Bersten A, Soni N, Oh TE (eds) (2003) Oh's intensive care manual, 5th edn. Oxford: Butterworth Heinemann.

Hough A (2001) Physiotherapy in respiratory care: a problem solving approach to respiratory and cardiac management, 3rd edn. Cheltenham: Stanley Thornes.

Pryor JA, Prasad SA (eds) (2002) Physiotherapy for respiratory and cardiac problems, 3rd edn. London: Churchill Livingstone.

Singer M, Webb A (eds) (2005) Oxford handbook of critical care, 2nd revised edn. Oxford: Oxford University Press.

10

CHAPTER 11

Calls to paediatric ICU (PICU)

Elaine Dhouieb

Paediatric intensive care covers a wide range of conditions and ages from premature neonates to 16-year-olds. Physiotherapists should be aware of continuing lung development into teenage years. Chest clearance should be used only where indicated. Careful assessment and discussion with medical and nursing staff is needed. Clinical signs may be much more discreet, especially in infants.

Intensive care units are high-technology, frightening places for most people. Take advantage of skilled medical and nursing staff for help and advice. It may be more difficult to gain the cooperation of a small child in treatment, and consent issues must also be considered. Parents will have 24-hour access and in most units will not be asked to leave during treatment. Their needs, fears and anxieties must also be considered. Tables 11.1–11.4 detail the aims of physiotherapy in the PICU, inappropriate calls to the PICU, common PICU issues and PICU treatment precautions, respectively.

CONDITIONS

Patients are admitted to PICU with a wide range of conditions. They may have a wide range of congenital or other underlying conditions to be considered (Table 11.5). A proportion of children have severe neurological conditions which predispose them to respiratory complications.

THE CALL OUT

- Information gathered will be similar to that in adult ICU.
- Work closely with the nursing staff; they are exceptionally skilled at handling sick children.
- Ask lots of questions (see Chapter 4).
- Never be afraid to ask for help.

Table 11.1 Aims of physiotherapy on PICU

Aims of treatment
● Remove secretions
● Re-inflate areas of atelectasis
● Reduce airflow obstruction
● Improve gas exchange
● Decrease work of breathing
● Prevention of respiratory compromise

Table 11.2 Inappropriate calls to PICU

Potentially inappropriate calls	
Inhaled foreign body	● Physiotherapy may move the object further down the bronchial tree; do not treat until the child has had bronchoscopy to remove ● Reassess and treat as appropriate
Epiglottitis, croup, stridor	● Unless the child is intubated physiotherapy techniques may increase swelling and compromise respiration ● After extubation do not treat for at least 2 hours or if there is significant stridor
Bronchiolitis	● In a self-ventilating infant with no other underlying condition physiotherapy does not add any benefit to good nursing care of positioning, hydration and suction ● The ventilated infant should be assessed and treated if indicated
Whooping cough/pertussis	● In the acute phase of paroxysmal coughing, physiotherapy can initiate coughing which may compromise the child ● Only treat if there are retained secretions and the child is paralysed and sedated ● May have retained secretions after acute phase
Extreme prematurity or low birthweight	● See Chapter 18

Table 11.3 Common issues on PICU

Airways	<ul><li>Uncuffed nasal ET tubes are usually used to prevent airway damage</li><li>These must be securely anchored to prevent accidental extubation or nasal trauma</li><li>If the tube is insecure, retaping or extreme caution is required</li></ul>
Mechanical ventilation	<ul><li>Be familiar with the ventilators used in your unit</li><li>Pressure-limiting ventilation is used to decrease the risk of barotrauma</li><li>In pressure ventilation, tidal volume will fall with decreased lung compliance, e.g. secretions (can be used as an outcome measure)</li></ul>
PEEP	<ul><li>PEEP is usually used to prevent airway closure</li><li>Must be maintained during manual hyperinflation</li></ul>
Oxygen	<ul><li>The risk of desaturation with physiotherapy and suction can be avoided if the child is pre-oxygenated by increasing FiO_2 by 10%</li><li>Check with nurses that this is appropriate</li><li>Infants should be hand-ventilated with an air/oxygen mix to prevent retinopathy of prematurity and lung oxygen toxicity</li><li>Weaning children who are making respiratory effort should be bagged with an air/oxygen mix to prevent loss of respiratory drive by blowing off too much CO_2</li></ul>
Inhaled nitric oxide (iNO)	<ul><li>This is used specifically to lower pulmonary arterial pressure (to improve lung compliance) without effect on systemic pressures</li><li>Patients must be hand-ventilated with the NO on and changeover from ventilator to bag should be quick to prevent swings in pulmonary arterial pressure</li><li>Closed suction or suction through the bagging system port should be used to prevent leakage</li><li>**If you are pregnant you may be advised not to treat patients receiving NO – check hospital policy**</li></ul>

Table 11.3 *Continued*

High-frequency oscillatory ventilation (HFOV)	● This ventilates by diffusion and is used where limits of conventional ventilation have been reached ● May prevent barotrauma ● As physiotherapy techniques including MHI work by changing pressure they are not indicated unless there are excess secretions and the patient is stable, or until the weaning phase ● **Check the unit policy before treating patients on HFOV** ● Positioning, humidification and suction are vital ● Closed-circuit suction is used to prevent loss of pressure
Extracorporeal membrane oxygenation (ECMO)	● This is used mainly in designated centres and may be useful especially in neonates ● If the lungs are being inflated it will be at low pressures ● Anticoagulants make the infant susceptible to bleeds, both pulmonary and cerebral ● Great care must be taken with lines when positioning as dislodgement could be potentially fatal
Weaning	● Weaning in infants is more gradual than in adults due to the anatomical and physiological differences (Chapter 4) ● Large amounts of dead space, e.g. in ventilator tubing, may increase work of breathing ● Patient may be weaned onto nasal short tube or mask CPAP
Bi-level positive airway pressure (BiPAP)	● Patients, especially with neuromuscular conditions, may be weaned from ventilation onto this via a mask or tracheostomy ● Also useful as an adjunct to chest clearance

Table 11.4 Treatment precautions on PICU

Positioning	• **Head-down position should not be used routinely** • Infants are particularly prone to reflux and as paediatric ET tubes are generally uncuffed there is no airway protection • Prone positioning decreases the work of breathing, improves gas exchange by stabilizing the anterior chest wall and improving V/Q matching, and is often used • **Because of the link with sudden infant death syndrome it should not be used in infants whose respiration is not monitored by ECG, pulse oximetry or mattress alarm** • Infants and children who are paralysed and sedated are much easier to move but glide sheets, etc. should still be used in the older child, both for their comfort and for staff • Great care must be taken not to damage joints and tissues especially in infants • Nesting and containment positioning are important developmentally for ventilated small infants
Percussion, shaking/vibration	• **In paralysed and sedated babies their heads should be stabilized to prevent shaking injury to the brain**
Manual hyperinflation (MHI)	• MHI correctly applied can be an efficient adjunct to chest clearance • In children up to 5 years old, open-ended bags are used to prevent overinflation • Infants are PEEP dependent, therefore it must be maintained • PEEP >7–10 mmHg can be difficult to replicate and MHI is not advised
Bronchoalveolar lavage (BAL)	• Can be diagnostic or an adjunct to physiotherapy • **Use if within your scope of practice and if trained in the technique** • May cause decreased lung compliance initially (patient may need increased ventilation post BAL) • May be effective in acute atelectasis or smoke inhalation in stable patient

11

Table 11.5 Conditions commonly seen on PICU

Head injury or cerebral oedema	<ul><li>See Chapter 14</li><li>Frequent in children</li><li>Aim is to prevent secondary injury</li><li>May have aspirated at injury</li><li>Meticulous assessment – is low CPP (MAP, ICP) caused by low BP, neurological (raised ICP) or retained secretions (raised CO_2)?</li><li>Use three people to treat (MHI, suction and physiotherapy), to prevent swings in CO_2</li><li>MHI may efficiently move secretions with no compromise of CPP</li><li>Slow percussion and rests between shaking to prevent stair step (increase then increase with no return to baseline), rise in ICP with increased pressure</li><li>Use end tidal CO_2 monitor in circuit</li><li>Assess and treat little but often</li><li>When able to turn, log roll to prevent kinking blood vessels reducing cerebral outflow</li><li>High risk of DVT; use pressure stockings</li></ul>
Cardiac surgery/cardiology	<ul><li>Surgery may be palliative (not normal anatomy or blood flow), staging (leading to complete repair) or correcting (normal anatomy and blood flow)</li><li>Be aware of change in anatomy and flows (too much or too little blood going to lungs)</li><li>Open sternum, paralysed, therefore at risk of chest problems</li><li>Some units treat patients with open chests with MHI and posterior vibrations; careful positioning, ¼ turn if indicated</li><li>Pulmonary hypertensive crisis – systemic circulation too low to be able to support rise in pulmonary pressure</li><li>May be caused by stress or intervention such as physiotherapy, suctioning or retained secretions – can lead to cardiac arrest</li><li>Careful treatment only if retained secretions; ensure adequate sedation and paralysis, monitor PA and systemic pressure. Acute treatment – hand bagging with 100% O_2</li><li>Phrenic nerve damage – raised diaphragm on CXR. Children particularly prone. Loss of lung volume, position head up to reduce work of breathing</li></ul>

11

Table 11.5 *Continued*

Tracheo-oesophageal fistula repair (congenital hole between trachea and oesophagus)	● May have tight repair ● No head extension as stretches suture line ● No MHI unless necessary to clear secretions or inflate atelectasis ● Careful measured length suction especially when extubated to prevent trauma to repair site
Gastroschisis/ exomphalos (abdominal contents outside wall)	● Distended abdomen ● No increase in intrathoracic pressure ● Care with manual techniques ● MHI – use only if absolutely essential and with caution due to increased pressure on abdomen
Congenital abnormalities of lung	● No MHI if cysts
Diaphragmatic hernia	● Hypoplastic lung on affected side ● No MHI
Spinal injury (see Chapter 14)	● Surgical repair more rare ● Very frightening for young child ● Less able to cope with respiratory compromise
Burns	● May use turning bed if artificial skin used (unable to use manual techniques) ● BAL if smoke inhalation ● Care with suction
Meningococcal septicaemia	● May be very unstable ● May be on haemofiltration ● May have pulmonary oedema or cerebral oedema
Non-accidental injury	● Usually head injury in PICU ● May have other injuries

11

Key messages

● Read through the other appropriate paediatric chapters (Chapters 1, 4, 17 and 19).
● Approach management of the PICU patient in the same systematic and logical format that you would use in any patient.
● Utilize the experience of the medical and nursing staff.
● Paediatric patients are more prone to atelectasis and retained secretions. They will fatigue and/or deteriorate more quickly – you will need to respond promptly.
● Always support a baby's head when performing manual techniques.
● Reflect and discuss your call out experiences.
● **Don't be scared!**

Further reading

Prasad SA, Hussey J (1995) Paediatric respiratory care, a guide for physiotherapists and health professionals. London: Chapman Hall.

Pryor JA, Webber BA 1998 Physiotherapy for respiratory and cardiac problems, 2nd edn. Edinburgh: Churchill Livingstone.

CHAPTER 12

Calls to the medical unit

Elizabeth Thomas

Medical patients regularly present with complicated multi-pathologies, often involving more than one system, each having a significant impact on the others. This chapter looks at some of the more common pathologies that the on call physiotherapist will encounter, highlighting important points to consider when assessing and treating the medical patient.

COPD

COPD exacerbations may be idiopathic or caused by bacterial or viral infection. Hypoxaemia will be the primary reason for the call out and the aim of physiotherapy is to establish the cause of hypoxaemia and treat as appropriate.

Major causes of hypoxaemia in COPD exacerbation include:

● Bronchospasm
● Sputum retention
● Consolidation.

Others common causes include:

● Cardiac event
● Pneumothorax
● Pulmonary embolus.

CONTROLLED OXYGEN THERAPY AND COPD

Oxygen is a drug and should be prescribed. Prescription should include percentage, flow rate, delivery device and whether oxygen delivery is intermittent or continuous. Any changes to oxygen therapy should be discussed with medical staff. Prescription may be flexible, for example 'maintain sats between 88% and 92%', in which case the FiO_2 can be changed as necessary until the desired saturation is reached.

NB: Liaise with medical staff to establish target SpO_2 levels for each individual patient. They may be as low as 80–85% in chronically hypoxic patients.

The role of the physiotherapist in relation to oxygen therapy includes:

● Assessment of oxygenation prior to, during and following treatment
● Ensuring the patient is receiving oxygen as prescribed

● Informing medical staff of increasing oxygen requirements
● Humidification of FiO_2 >30% (or lower if secretions are tenacious).

Some patients with COPD are classified as oxygen sensitive and have a chronically raised $PaCO_2$. They rely on a low PaO_2 to stimulate breathing, rather than an altered pH. This is called *hypoxic drive*. If too much oxygen is given, their stimulus to breathe (low PaO_2) is removed and the patient stops breathing, resulting in type II respiratory failure, sometimes called *oxygen-induced respiratory acidosis*.

It is vital that all COPD patients receive *controlled oxygen therapy* until it is established whether they are oxygen sensitive (through arterial blood gas analysis).

BEST PRACTICE FOR INITIAL USE OF SUPPLEMENTAL OXYGEN THERAPY IN COPD (NICE 2004)

● Maintain adequate O_2 levels (saturations ≥90%) without precipitating respiratory acidosis or worsening hypercapnia.
● Deliver O_2 via a controlled system such as a Venturi device. If a mask is not tolerated O_2 may be delivered via nasal cannulae.
● Until it is established whether a COPD patient is O_2 sensitive, start FiO_2 at 0.28 and increase until PaO_2 is >7.6 kPa, without causing a significant fall in pH.
● The COPD patient with respiratory acidosis, despite optimal medical management and controlled oxygen therapy, will require NIV or IPPV.
● If the COPD patient is not O_2 sensitive, increase FiO_2 until saturations are ≥90%.

MANAGEMENT OF THE COPD PATIENT WITH RESPIRATORY ACIDOSIS REQUIRING NIV (BRITISH THORACIC SOCIETY STANDARDS OF CARE COMMITTEE 2002)

(Refer to Chapter 9.)
● Only consider NIV following optimal medical management and controlled O_2 therapy.
● COPD patients are at risk of pneumothorax with positive pressure ventilation.
● Use controlled O_2 therapy when removing from NIV.

CAUSES OF READMISSION IN COPD

Physiotherapy can play an important role in establishing the cause of frequent admissions in some patients and in helping to prevent such admissions (Table 12.1).

CARE OF THE PATIENT WITH END-STAGE COPD

It is important to establish the ceiling of treatment agreed by the patient, their family and their medical team. IPPV may be deemed futile, and the fully informed

Table 12.1 Common causes of readmission in the COPD patient

Cause	Advice
Uncontrolled symptoms	● Optimize medical therapy ● Shortness of breath ● Teach techniques for mastery of breathlessness ● Assess need for short-burst or ambulatory oxygen therapy ● Sputum retention ● Assist sputum clearance without impacting on breathlessness ● Consider whether mucolytics may be beneficial
Recurrent need for NIV	● Patients with late-stage COPD may require domiciliary NIV to prevent relapse into type II respiratory failure
Anxiety or depression	● Be alert to depression in COPD patients who are hypoxic (SpO_2 <92%), have severe dyspnoea, or have been admitted with exacerbation

patient may decide that NIV is not in their best interest; treatment may consist solely of medications and physiotherapy.

Assess the patient and formulate your plan and goals in line with what the patient wishes to achieve. There may be some disparity between what you perceive as optimal treatment and what the patient consents to. Some patients may wish to limit treatment to symptom control while others may feel that any intervention will worsen shortness of breath, outweighing any benefits gained, and thus decline what physiotherapy has to offer. These patients, who have had years of coping with unpleasant and disabling symptoms and have often had multiple inpatient admissions, are able to make truly informed choices.

Patients with end-stage COPD, together with their families and carers, should have access to the full range of services offered by the multidisciplinary palliative care teams, including admission to hospices. Opioids, benzodiazepines, tricyclic antidepressants and oxygen therapy may be used for the palliation of breathlessness in patients unresponsive to other medical treatments. In the terminal stages of the disease, antisecretory agents may be useful.

ACUTE ASTHMA

Optimal medical management is essential during acute exacerbation of asthma and may include magnesium infusion, inhaled or nebulized bronchodilators (beta-2 agonists and antimuscarinics), inhaled, nebulized, oral or intravenous corticosteroids, and theophyllines. Antibiotics will be used if there is evidence of infection (↑white cell count, neutrophils and CRP, ± pyrexia) (Table 12.2).

Table 12.2 Common issues in the treatment of patients with acute asthma

Common issues	Advice
Bronchospasm	● Be calm ● Ensure adequate, humidified O_2. Heated humidification may be necessary. Cold water humidification may exacerbate bronchospasm ● Treat ½ hour post bronchodilators if possible ● Re-assess regularly and discontinue treatment if bronchospasm worsens ● ACBT ● Avoid repeated huffing or coughing – it may worsen bronchospasm ● Emphasize periods of breathing control ● Remember manual techniques may ↑ bronchospasm
Sputum plugs Sticky plugs or casts of sputum are common. These may cause plugging off of major airways, leading to lobar collapse	● Ensure O_2 is humidified ● Consider mucolytics ● Encourage oral or i.v. fluids if patient shows signs of dehydration ● Slow, single-handed percussion may be useful providing it does not increase bronchospasm ● See Chapter 6
The tiring patient Inspiratory _and_ expiratory polyphonic wheeze or a silent chest on auscultation are signs of deteriorating asthma Beware of 'normal' blood gases. Initially patients show type I respiratory failure ± hypocapnia. As they tire, pCO_2 rises, but ABGs may have been taken as pCO_2 is rising through the normal range. Look for signs of CO_2 retention/narcosis (see Chapter 9)	● If you suspect the patient is deteriorating, ask for an urgent medical review ● Use positioning to optimize respiratory muscle function and reduce work of breathing ● Only use sputum clearance techniques if you think sputum retention is significant in causing airway obstruction (refer to Chapter 6) ● Avoid tiring patient further. Restrict to short, regular treatments ● Non-invasive or invasive ventilation will be required for patients with type 2 respiratory failure (refer to Chapter 9) ● _! NB: Check for pneumothorax before applying non-invasive ventilation_ (refer to CXR and auscultation sections)

PANCREATITIS

Pancreatitis can be acute (one-off occurrence), chronic where it persists even after the cause has been removed, or hereditary. Causes include gallstones, excessive alcohol consumption, hypertriglyceridaemia, viral infection, trauma, vasculitis or pregnancy.

The aim of physiotherapy is to identify and treat the cause of hypoxaemia (Table 12.3).

TREATMENT OF THE RENAL PATIENT

Renal failure is characterized by raised urea and creatinine levels. Electrolytes may also become deranged (Tables 12.4, 12.5 and 12.6).

OESOPHAGEAL VARICES

Oesophageal varices are extremely dilated submucosal veins in the oesophagus. They are a consequence of portal hypertension as seen in liver cirrhosis. They are very likely to bleed and are diagnosed via endoscopy (Table 12.7).

INTERSTITIAL LUNG DISEASE

Interstitial lung disease (ILD) refers to a group of lung diseases characterized by inflammation which often leads to pulmonary fibrosis. Fibrosis destroys the alveoli, interstitium and capillary network of the affected areas of lung resulting in a restrictive disorder (Table 12.8).

Table 12.3 Common issues in the management of the medical patient with pancreatitis

Common issues/complications	Advice
Pain Severe upper abdominal pain radiating to the back causing ↓TV and atelectasis Opiates may reduce respiratory drive Lobar or lung collapse is common as a consequence of upper abdominal pain NB: ↓BS may be due to pleural effusion, also commonly seen in pancreatitis (see sections on respiratory assessment and CXR)	● Ensure adequate analgesia prior to treatment ● Check respiratory rate. If <12 b.p.m., discuss alternative forms of analgesia with team ● See Chapter 7
Distended abdomen Limits diaphragmatic excursion leading to volume loss	● Position patient to allow free movement of diaphragm ● See Chapter 7

Table 12.3 *Continued*

Common issues/complications	Advice
Hypoxaemia As a consequence of: Volume loss Acute pneumonitis Pancreatic enzymes may directly damage the lungs ARDS SIRS and multi-organ dysfunction syndrome are known complications of pancreatitis. Signs and symptoms of ARDS include $\uparrow O_2$ requirement, hypoxaemia refractory to O_2 therapy, tachypnoea and non-cardiogenic pulmonary oedema Aspiration pneumonia Vomiting is common with pancreatitis. Look for signs of sudden respiratory distress following a history of vomiting. Often affects the right middle or lower lobe	● See Chapter 7 ● May require high-flow, heated humidified O_2 therapy. CPAP may be indicated ● Physiotherapy cannot improve the underlying process, but assess for sputum retention and use positioning to alleviate SOB/$\downarrow$WOB ● Humidify high-flow oxygen ● CPAP may be indicated ● Patients commonly require intubation and ventilation ● Physiotherapy is of limited benefit ● *Prompt treatment will limit pneumonitis* ● Use postural drainage if appropriate, manual techniques and ACBT to mobilize aspirate. Clear with FET, cough or suction
Dehydration Common as a result of vomiting and internal bleeding	● Assess fluid balance and observation charts. Urea will be raised (with normal creatinine) in the dehydrated patient (see glossary of normal values) ● Electrolyte disturbance is possible with vomiting. Check blood results prior to treatment ● Ensure CVS stability prior to treatment ● Humidify O_2 therapy
Sepsis ARDS is a manifestation of SIRS	● Look for cardiovascular implications of sepsis – low BP, high HR ● Report worsening signs of sepsis/ARDS: Increasing O_2 requirement or RR, decreasing BP or increasing HR, cardiovascular instability. Use early warning system, e.g. MEWS, if utilized by your Trust

Table 12.4 Common issues in the management of the patient with renal failure

Common issues	Advice
Tachypnoea May be due to respiratory compensation of metabolic acidosis Acute renal failure may result in oliguria leading to CCF, pulmonary oedema and pleural effusions	● Physiotherapy is of limited benefit unless there is evidence of co-existing respiratory complications
Tenacious sputum Renal patients may be fluid restricted and will be receiving diuretic therapy/dialysis	● Humidify O_2 ● Encourage fluids if allowed
Altered mental state/confusion/seizures Altered mental state may be due to hypoxaemia, deranged electrolytes or changes in pH	● Assess whether SpO_2 is low ● Ensure O_2 is delivered as prescribed ● Liaise with medical staff if O_2 requirement increased ● May be difficult to gain informed consent. Treat in patient's best interest

Table 12.5 Common issues when treating the patient with chronic or acute-on-chronic renal failure

Common issues	Advice
Osteoporosis	● Check CXR for signs of fractures ● Ensure adequate analgesia prior to treatment ● Care with manual techniques
Anaemia	● Check Hb prior to treatment (refer to glossary of normal values in Appendix 2) ● Patients may be tissue hypoxic with normal SaO_2 ● May contribute to breathlessness
↓Immune response/↓WCC	● ↑risk of opportunistic infection ● Use reverse barrier methods in line with hospital protocol

12

Table 12.6 Causes of cardiovascular instability in the patient with renal failure

Cause	Advice
Electrolyte disturbance (risk of arrhythmia)	● Check K^+ and Ca^{++} levels prior to treatment (refer to glossary of normal values in Appendix 2) ● If deranged, check imbalance is being treated or contact the team
Cardiac tamponade and pericarditis	● Establish diagnosis from notes ● Examine observation charts and ensure CVS stability prior to treatment ● Liaise with nursing staff regarding response to handling
Patients on haemofiltration may be CVS unstable due to rapid changes in fluid status	● Examine observation charts ● Liaise with nursing staff

Table 12.7 Common issues when treating patients with oesophageal varices

Common issues	Advice
Actively bleeding oesophageal varices	● **All physiotherapy is contraindicated**
Deranged clotting	● **Suction is contraindicated** ● Care with manual techniques and coughing ● Utilize ACBT with huffing, positioning and mobilization to assist sputum clearance and prevent respiratory complications **NB: Do not use postural drainage or positive pressure treatments with these patients**
Treated oesophageal varices	● **Suction and postural drainage remain contraindicated**

PNEUMONIA

Pneumonia results from an inflammation of the alveolar space, usually due to invasion by bacteria, viruses or fungi, or as a result of chemical or physical injury. In bacterial and fungal infection, alveoli fill with protein-rich fluid and debris from white blood cells. Sputum production also increases (Table 12.9).

Interstitial pneumonia is characterized by patchy or diffuse inflammation of the interstitium (the area between the alveoli). The alveoli do *not* contain significant exudate.

Table 12.8 Common issues when treating patients with pulmonary fibrosis

Common issues	Advice
Dry, irritating cough	● Physiotherapy is not indicated unless there is a superimposed respiratory tract infection
Fatigue	● Discuss energy conservation and pacing
SOB Profoundly ↓lung compliance in fibrotic lung disease causes extreme SOB on exertion and eventually at rest. It can be extremely distressing	● Reassure +++ ● Teach positions of ease to optimize respiratory muscle function and reduce WOB ● Pharmaceutical palliation of breathlessness is necessary in end-stage disease (see palliative care for COPD patient above)
Severe hypoxaemia At rest: Fibrosis slows diffusion of O_2 across the respiratory membrane (diffusion defect)	● Ensure adequate FiO_2 is being delivered by monitoring SpO_2 ● Keep O_2 mask on throughout treatment ● Humidify FiO_2 >30% ● CPAP is often required to maintain oxygenation ● If type II respiratory failure develops, NIV or invasive ventilation will be required, if appropriate **NB: Higher pressures will be required to ventilate 'stiff lungs' so ↑risk of pneumothorax**
On exertion: Exertion speeds up pulmonary blood flow resulting in even less time for Hb to be oxygenated. This can cause extreme dips in SpO_2	● Monitor SpO_2 closely during treatment ● Always ensure adequate O_2 delivery when moving the fibrotic patient. An ↑FiO_2 will probably be required ● Dips in SpO_2 and breathlessness on exertion will resolve with rest and O_2 therapy. Be patient. It may take several minutes

CYSTIC FIBROSIS (ADULT)

Adult cystic fibrosis (CF) patients will have their own independent airway clearance regime. It may comprise of PD ± self-percussion and ACBT, PEP mask, Flutter device or the Acapella. You do not need to be an expert in all these techniques, but during infective exacerbation you need to assess the effectiveness of the normal regime, and assist with sputum clearance if necessary. Patients may benefit from PD and manual techniques performed by the physiotherapist. It is advisable to do one or two lung areas with each treatment. Treatment may need to be further modified in the patient with dyspnoea, e.g. modified PD, ↑emphasis on breathing control (Association of Chartered Physiotherapists in Cystic Fibrosis 2002) (Table 12.10).

Table 12.9 Management of patients with pneumonia

Type of pneumonia	Advice
Bronchopneumonia Typically caused by bacteria Consolidation is patchy involving one or more lobes, usually dependent lung zones. Exudate (consolidation) is centred in the bronchi and bronchioles with spread to adjacent alveoli. May progress to lobar pneumonia Aspiration causes an initial pneumonitis which often leads to bronchopneumonia RML and RLL are most commonly affected. Prompt removal of aspirate will limit pneumonitis and the risk of bacterial pneumonia	● Ensure adequate, humidified O_2 therapy ● Use sputum clearance techniques including ACBT, manual techniques and positioning as indicated ● Consider saline nebulizers or mucolytics if sputum tenacious ● Use chest X-ray to determine affected lobes. Use PD to drain the affected areas. *Remember each lobe has several segments* ● Consider suction or cough-assist in those patients unable to cough effectively
Lobar/multilobar pneumonia Consolidation in one or more lobes Typically caused by bacterial infection	● Ensure adequate, humidified O_2 therapy ● Position to optimize V/Q matching and therefore arterial oxygenation (down with the good lung in unilateral disease) ● Further physiotherapy is not indicated in non-productive, fully consolidated pneumonia ● Re-assess daily and use sputum clearance techniques if patient has a productive cough. See Chapter 6
Interstitial pneumonia Often caused by viruses or atypical bacteria. Viral pneumonia may make patient more susceptible to superimposed bacterial pneumonia	● Physiotherapy not indicated unless evidence of bacterial infection
Fungal pneumonia Commonly affects immunosuppressed patients. Includes *Pneumocystis jiroveci* (previously called *P. carinii* pneumonia or PCP).	● Ensure O_2 therapy is humidified ● Position to ↓WOB ● Severely hypoxaemic patients will require CPAP

12

Table 12.9 *Continued*

Type of pneumonia	Advice
Can cause extreme hypoxaemia and rapid onset of type I and II respiratory failure. Non-productive in early stages	● Patients in type II respiratory failure will require NIV or IPPV ● Further physiotherapy not indicated unless evidence of sputum retention ● You may be asked for an induced sputum specimen for diagnosis of *P. jiroveci*. This is not an on call procedure
Pandemic pneumonia Includes: SARS (severe acute respiratory syndrome), caused by the coronavirus Highly contagious and mortality is high Last seen in China in 2003 Primary viral pneumonia and secondary bacterial pneumonia as a consequence of pandemic influenza	● Follow your local hospital infection control guidelines for pandemic pneumonia ● Only treat those patients who have evidence of sputum retention. Treat as presents, i.e. bronchopneumonia or lobar pneumonia (see above)

Table 12.10 Common issues in the treatment of adult CF patients

Common issues	Advice
Haemoptysis Blood streaking Moderate haemoptysis Frank haemoptysis	● Treat as normal ● Use TEEs and gentle huffing only. Minimize coughing ● Discontinue physiotherapy until bleeding settles. Humidify O_2
Type I respiratory failure Hypoxaemic episodes will become more common as disease progresses	● Ensure adequate, humidified O_2 therapy. Heated humidification may be necessary with thick secretions ● Effective sputum clearance will decrease airway obstruction and improve oxygenation. Check SpO_2 pre and post treatment ● Monitor SpO_2 and modify treatment if it causes significant dips, e.g. modify PD positions, limit periods of huffing, ↑emphasis on breathing control, salbutamol nebulizer pre or post treatment

12

Table 12.10 *Continued*

Common issues	Advice
Type II respiratory failure NIV may be used as a bridge to lung or heart/lung transplant. Patients may have domiciliary NIV (for overnight use or more prolonged periods) and are likely to be confident with its use	● NIV or IPPV will be required for patients in type II respiratory failure ● Treat patients on NIV with their mask on, removing it to allow expectoration ● A nasal mask may be more suitable for those with copious secretions ● Monitor saturations throughout treatment ● This should not influence physiotherapy management ● **NB: CF patients have an ↑risk of pneumothorax with positive pressure techniques** (See Chapters 5 and 19)
Infection control	● Always treat patients with MRSA, *Pseudomonas aeruginosa* or *Burkholderia cepacia* last if possible ● Ensure strict hand hygiene and follow local hospital guidelines for infection control
Osteoporosis CF patients often have poor uptake of vitamin D which can lead to osteoporosis	● Use caution with manual techniques ● Ensure adequate pain relief prior to treatment if necessary
Liver disease This is common in the later stages of CF Ascites will impinge on the diaphragm causing volume loss Liver disease may cause portal hypertension leading to oesophageal varices	● Position patient to allow free movement of the diaphragm (see Chapter 7) ● These patients will not tolerate head-down tilts ● Treatment with the Acapella, Flutter device or PEP mask may be more appropriate ● See previous section on oesophageal varices
Terminal stages of CF Not all patients want, or are suitable for, transplant. This is an extremely distressing time for both the patient and their family. Patients should have access to bereavement counsellors and the palliative care team who will manage their symptoms	● Treat for comfort only, at the patient's request

BRONCHIECTASIS

Bronchiectasis is the abnormal dilatation of bronchi caused by destruction of muscular and elastic components of the bronchial walls. The airways lose their normal sputum clearance mechanisms. Causes include TB, pertussis, measles, aspiration of a foreign body or severe bacterial pneumonia (often in childhood). It is an obstructive lung disease and usually affects one or more lobes (commonly the lower lobes). Signs and symptoms include chronic purulent sputum production (sometimes several cupfuls a day), regular and often persistent respiratory tract infections, chronic cough, disturbed sleep, fatigue and finger clubbing. Bronchiectatic patients, like CF patients, usually have their own airway clearance regime. It may comprise of PD ± self-percussion and ACBT, PEP mask, Flutter device or the Acapella (see CF section above). In acute infective exacerbation they may require assistance to achieve effective sputum clearance. Common issues include type I respiratory failure, haemoptysis and infection control (see Table 12.10). In the later stages of the disease, patients may admit with type II respiratory failure requiring NIV or IPPV (see Chapter 9).

References

Association of Chartered Physiotherapists in Cystic Fibrosis (2002) Clinical guidelines for the physiotherapy management of cystic fibrosis. www.cftrust.org.uk.

British Thoracic Society Standards of Care Committee (2002) Non-invasive ventilation in acute respiratory failure. Thorax 57:192–211.

National Institute for Clinical Excellence (2004) Chronic obstructive pulmonary disease: management of chronic obstructive pulmonary disease in adults in primary and secondary care. www.nice.org.uk/CG012NICEguideline.

Further reading

West JB (1995) Respiratory physiology: the essentials, 5th edn. London: Williams and Wilkins.

West JB (1995) Pulmonary pathophysiology: the essentials, 5th edn. London: Williams and Wilkins.

12

CHAPTER 13

Calls to the surgical ward

Valerie Ball and Mary-Ann Broad

This chapter covers:
- Considerations in the assessment of the surgical patient
- Calls to a general surgery patient
- Calls to vascular, orthopaedic, plastic, ENT and maxillofacial surgery patients
- Calls to theatre/recovery room
- Calls to the ward-based tracheostomy patient.

CONSIDERATIONS IN THE ASSESSMENT OF A SURGERY PATIENT

| Be Aware! | It is key to find out the type, reason and date of surgery. Determine the extent of the incision. |

CNS
- Type and effectiveness of pain control – is analgesia sufficient for full assessment and treatment?
- Major abdominal surgery is often associated with high levels of pain. This can impact on the function of the diaphragm and inhibit the patient from moving or coughing. Adequate patient analgesia is vital to assess the patient and perform an effective treatment.

Cardiovascular system
What is the patient's rate/rhythm? Is it compromising their blood pressure? See Appendix 2 for normal values.
- **High blood pressure** may be caused by:
  - Pain/anxiety
  - Uncontrolled hypertension.
- **Low blood pressure** may be caused by:
  - Dehydration
  - Postoperative bleeding

- Sepsis
- Epidural analgesia.
- What effect is your treatment likely to have on this?
- **Pyrexia >38.5°C for >8 hours** can be due to a lower respiratory tract infection. NB: Surgery may cause reflex pyrexia – temperature gradually rises and falls within 24 hours of operation; this change in temperature is not due to infection.
- A raised white blood cell count will confirm infection (WCC >12 × 10^9/L). NB: WCC may not rise in elderly patients.

Renal/fluid balance

- Input:
  - Is oral intake allowed?
  - Is i.v. fluid being given?
- Output: Normal urine output = 1 ml/kg/hour, i.e. a 60-kg woman should pass 60 ml of urine each hour. Include wound drains and insensible loss (sweat and loss of fluid from respiratory tract and GI tract = 1 litre/day).
- Positive balance (input > output). A positive fluid balance may give some signs that can be confused with secretion retention; therefore consider the following. Causes of a positive balance may include:
  - Left ventricular failure
  - Cardiac arrhythmia
  - Renal failure
  - Profound malnutrition.
  Look for other signs of fluid retention before assuming a positive balance is fluid overload, i.e.:
  When calculating consider:
  - Blood loss in theatre
  - A recent history of vomiting and or diarrhoea
  - Insensible loss increases by approximately 1 litre of fluid for each °C per day above 37°C.
  Remember that pulmonary oedema can co-exist with a respiratory tract infection in the severely ill patient.
  - Peripheral pitting oedema (sacral oedema in bed-bound patients)
  - Raised JVP
  - Frothy sputum
  - Dependent fine crackles on auscultation.
- Negative balance (output > input). Dehydration may be contributing to a sputum retention problem.

Respiratory system

Respiratory rate

- Low (<10) – if due to morphine overdose, the patient will often have pinpoint pupils which may require reversal, e.g. Narcan (naloxone hydrochloride). Inform ward staff immediately.
- High (>20) – indicates cardiorespiratory compromise (perhaps due to pain, V/Q mismatch, cardiac or renal problem, etc.); a careful assessment is required.
- Very high (>35) – very severe problem.

Respiratory pattern

- Are there chest drains in situ? What are they there for?
- Is the respiratory pattern limited by pain or thoracic stiffness?

ABGs

A small deterioration in PaO_2 is normal in the first 24 hours post abdominal surgery.

- Very prolonged procedure (5 hours or more) or major blood replacement (5 units or more) are risk factors for ARDS developing 2–3 days post surgery. Deteriorating ABGs despite increasing FiO_2 may signal its onset.

Oxygen therapy and SpO_2

Oxygen therapy is usually prescribed for 24–48 hours post surgery. Aim to keep **SpO_2 >95%** to reduce the risks of delayed healing, infection and confusion. It is important to make sure O_2 is appropriately humidified. Patients with pre-existing cardiopulmonary disease may have **nocturnal dips** in SpO_2 for 5 days after surgery. Patients often have oxygen delivered by a simple face mask but these masks are only suitable for delivery of between 40% and 60% O_2 as below 5 L/min delivery CO_2 retention can occur. Use a Venturi system (high-flow mask with accurate oxygen delivery) or nasal cannula to deliver higher or lower concentrations (see Chapter 9).

Mobilization

Any limits to mobility (especially in specialist units – see sections below). Consider:

- Drips/drains/lines
- CVS stability/reserve
- Respiratory reserve
- Contraindications, e.g. unstable CVS.

Drug chart

If **nil by mouth (NBM)**, the patient may not have received their usual medication, which can cause problems as diverse as there are drugs, e.g. a rheumatoid patient may be more immobile.

CALLS TO A GENERAL SURGERY PATIENT
Introduction

This section will concentrate on the problems commonly met by patients having a major abdominal incision, see Appendix 3. The patient may be nursed on a surgical ward or on a high-dependency unit, but the principles of management are the same.

Common problems in the post-surgical patient:
- Pain
- Unibasal or bibasal atelectasis
- Sputum retention.

Pain

Check drug chart for type/timing of medication. Ask patient to move in bed or take a deep breath for more accurate assessment of pain control; if they can do this then most treatment techniques are possible. Ideally they should be able to move freely in bed.

> **KEY POINT**
> Ensure analgesia is optimized prior to your arrival on the ward.

Analgesia options
Opiates (e.g. morphine)
- Affects the CNS, causing drowsiness and potentially respiratory depression.

Epidurals
- Require less morphine for the same level of analgesia; some include a local anaesthetic. Patients tend to be less drowsy or nauseous with this method.
- Nursing staff (within set parameters) can adjust dosage. If not effective over the appropriate dermatomes needs replacing with an alternative from list below.
- NOT to be disconnected. Careful handling required to avoid dislodging fine-bore tube from spinal insertion.

- Can result in sensory/motor loss in lower limbs limiting mobilization – check limb sensation/movement and use a walking frame for transfers/ standing providing arm strength is adequate and safe to do so.
- They can cause hypotension.

PCA (patient-controlled analgesia) and PCEA (patient-controlled epidural analgesia)
- IV infusion self administered by patient pressing handset, instruct how to use it a minute or two before moving/coughing. ONLY patient may press handset to self-administer morphine.
- Nurses will set a 'lock out period' when patient cannot receive a dose when pressing handset to prevent overdosing.

Intramuscular morphine
- Given as required (p.r.n.) as a 4–6-hourly injection; poor pain control as does not give continuous pain relief – discuss alternatives with medical team if contributing to problem.
- NB: i.v. analgesia will work almost immediately; i.m. or oral will take up to 30 minutes to take effect.

Uncontrolled pain
If no improvement and patient still unable to deep-breathe due to pain after analgesia – you may need to discuss this with an anaesthetist or make an urgent referral to the pain team.

Unibasal or bibasal atelectasis
Functional residual capacity (FRC) is reduced following abdominal surgery due to a multitude of causes, e.g. pain, effect of anaesthetic. The impact is basal atelectasis. Good pain management and positioning is key. For specific management see Chapter 7 on reduced lung volumes.

Sputum retention
Pain, drying of airways from O_2 therapy, inadequate fluid replacement and NBM notices all contribute to sputum retention. Causes need to be addressed to optimize treatment. Good pain management and appropriate humidification are key. For specific management see Chapter 6.

Other issues
- **Slumped position** is the most common position in which to find the abdominal surgery patient. Good use of pillows will ensure patient does not move back down after you leave the bedside. Sit patient out of bed as soon as stable.

● **Distended abdomen +/− paralytic ileus.** Frequently leads to bibasal atelectasis, position in high side-lying. Request medical review to establish cause.

GENERAL SURGERY TREATMENT PRECAUTIONS
● Increasing anxiety and pain
  ● Gaining trust from your patient is vital.
  ● Explain the rationale behind your treatment, that **some discomfort is to be expected when coughing or moving** and that you are going to do as much as possible to minimize this.
  ● Give the patient as much self-control as possible and **be supportive and careful when moving** or handling them.

TREATMENT CONTRAINDICATIONS
● Do not use postural drainage (head-down tip) after gastrectomy and oesophagogastrectomy.
● If cardiac (upper sphincter) of stomach has been removed, anastomosis and remaining oesophagus may be damaged by backflow of acid.

TREATMENT EXTREME CAUTIONS
● **ALWAYS** get consultant approval if IPPB or suctioning is required for a gastrectomy or oesophagectomy patient.
● Due to the position of the anastomosis, increased pressure or a suction catheter may cause damage.

CALLS TO OTHER SURGICAL AREAS

Be Aware! Being called to some non-general surgical ward areas may pose additional problems. These wards may not be used to dealing with patients who have respiratory compromise. You may need to advise staff in the basic management, e.g.:
● Positioning
● Oxygen therapy
● Humidification.

Vascular surgery unit
Peripheral vascular disease (PVD)
Often associated with ischaemic heart disease (IHD), cerebral degeneration and COPD; adjust treatment to individual needs.

Aortic aneurysm
Breathlessness and 'bubbly chest' may be a result of renal failure. This must be suspected if the aorta was clamped above the renal arteries during the operation; check the patient notes.

Arterial bypass graft
- Viability – is the graft functioning?
- Observe when positioning/moving patient for signs of:
  - Haemorrhage
  - Thrombosis
  - Nerve injury causing sensory/motor impairment
  - Ischaemia below graft site
- Discuss whether mobility is allowed with medical staff.

Femoro-popliteal bypass
Often long incision to access arteries above and below knee; some units may have restrictions on postoperative knee flexion.

13

TREATMENT CONTRAINDICATIONS
Axillo-femoral bypass
Manual chest clearance techniques are contraindicated over the side of the graft as it passes subcutaneously across the chest wall.

Orthopaedic surgery unit
Osteoporosis and hip fracture
A kyphotic chest may indicate collapsed thoracic vertebrae; the restricted chest movement this causes makes this mainly elderly female group of patients highly susceptible to pneumonia when immobile.
- Positioning these patients is challenging, often requiring a compromise between comfort and effectiveness.
- Sitting out of bed/mobilizing must be instituted as early as possible.
- Manual techniques should be viewed with extreme caution.

Replacement joint dislocation

Discuss with surgeon cost/benefit of positioning for optimal respiratory function. For example, to achieve forward-lean sitting, the hip may need to be flexed to >90° or in high side-lying the hip may be in an adducted position. Both of these instances increase the risk of dislocation.

External fixators

● Discuss with surgeon any limits to movement.
● Positioning a limb with a fixator when requiring side-lying is usually possible by protecting the other limb with pillows.
● Patients with pelvic fixators may have to remain supine; physiotherapists have to rely on good instruction in breathing exercises or mechanical adjuncts, e.g. IPPB to treat effectively.

Rib/sternal injuries

See Chapter 15.

Spinal injuries

See Chapter 14.

Plastic surgery unit

Dependent on site of graft there may be restrictions to movement and manual chest clearance techniques – discuss with surgeon the cost/benefit <u>before</u> commencing treatment.

In all situations be aware of local management guidelines and contra-indications/cautions to treatment.

KEY POINTS

● **No** manual techniques over any type of graft affecting the chest (split skin, pedicle or free flap).
● **Do not** change position or treat if you are unsure. ALWAYS seek advice from senior members of the team.
● *If you spot anything you think has changed or does not look correct please hand it over – you may be the first to notice a problem!*

ENT and oromaxillofacial surgery unit

There are a number of surgeries that can be undertaken in this field but those that are likely to cause respiratory compromise are detailed below.

Laryngectomy

Many of these patients have a preoperative history of smoking, alcohol abuse and/or malnutrition making this patient group a high-risk category for post-operative pulmonary complications.

- There will be a tracheostomy tube in place immediately after surgery <u>BUT</u> it is an end stoma – i.e. there is no connection to nose or mouth and thus is the patient's only airway! NB: Tracheostomy tube may be sutured in place. This will often then be replaced with a stoma button (Fig. 13.1).

- Patients may retain secretions and have some postoperative bloody secretions. These are common and need to be cleared – ACBT and FET work well.

- It is preferable to get the patient to self-expectorate and clear with a tissue. It is possible to suction down the stoma but check with local policy first.

> **TREATMENT EXTREME CAUTION**
> Never suction the tube or stoma with a Yankeur – you would block off the airway!

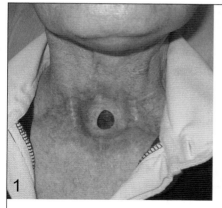
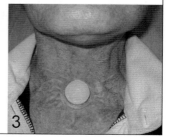
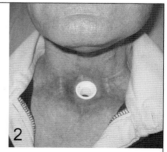

Laryngectomy Stoma

1 - Stoma (note blue voice prosthesis)
2 - Stoma button in situ
3 - HME

Figure 13.1 A stoma with and without a stoma button and HME.

● Ensure appropriate humidification, as all natural defences are lost; the patient is at risk of developing thick and sticky secretions. Think about oxygen delivery and appropriate methods of humidification. Some units use an HME (heat moisture exchanger) straight after surgery (see Fig. 13.1).

For management of tracheostomy patients, see below.

Facial/intra-oral reconstruction

This type of surgery may involve a free flap and takes place in specialist centres. You should be aware of your local guidelines in the management of these patients.

KEY POINTS
- **Do** keep head in midline to avoid kinking or tension on flap.
- **Do** avoid pressure from ETT tapes and trachy ties – if they are too tight they will compromise the flap.
- **Do** monitor chest closely as these patients are at high risk of postoperative complications.
- **Do not** perform manual techniques over the site of a new flap.
- **Do not** use Yankeur suction near an intra-oral flap – you may damage the flap.
- **Do not** change position or treat if you are unsure. ALWAYS seek advice from senior members of the team.

The speed at which complications are recognized is in direct proportion to the chances of survival of the flap. If you spot any changes or have any concerns please highlight them!

Communication issues

Postoperative swelling of the mouth and tongue is common and may hamper communication. If possible ascertain whether the patient had communication or literacy difficulties pre surgery.

Check whether the patient can see, hear, understand, use facial expression such as smile/blink, or write. It may be necessary to have established a method for the patient to indicate YES and NO – for example eye blink system, or have a picture/word/letter chart available.

CALLS TO THEATRE/RECOVERY

You may be called to recovery to a patient who has aspirated gastric contents at intubation/extubation or who has become very productive post surgery.

The theatre recovery room is rarely well stocked in basic therapy equipment; you will usually find airways, yankeurs, some suction catheters and protective gloves/aprons, etc. You may need to take with you oxygen and humidification equipment.

KEY POINTS
- Often a lack of appropriate oxygen +/– humidification equipment available.
- Postural drainage may be difficult/inappropriate if patient is still on a trolley – arrange to transfer to a bed if possible.
- It may be appropriate to suction the patient immediately. Theatre and recovery staff will be able to help you in setting up for this.
- Do not be afraid to ask staff on the unit to help – they will be very pleased to see you!

CALLS TO A WARD-BASED TRACHEOSTOMY PATIENT

Be Aware! NHS Trusts vary in the type/manufacturer of tracheostomy tubes used and the local protocol of tracheostomy care; this section is based on common themes from a number of Trusts in the UK. You need to be familiar with your local protocols before commencing on call duties.

Methods of tracheostomy tube insertion
For methods of tracheostomy tube insertion see Table 13.1.

Table 13.1 Methods of tracheostomy insertion

Surgical tracheostomy	Percutaneous tracheostomy	Mini-tracheostomy
Performed in theatre	Performed by dilation technique at bedside in ICU	Can be performed on any unit – but high risk of bleeding
Window in trachea – relatively stable	Window not stable – will close very quickly if tube removed in first 7–10 days and may not be possible to reinsert tube if comes out during this time	Window will not remain patent if removed. Can only be used for suction

Indications for a tracheostomy
- Emergency airway
  - Oral or nasal intubation impossible
- Trauma
  - Facial fractures
- Airway oedema
  - Burns
  - Drug sensitivities
  - Post ENT surgery
- Need for artificial ventilation >7 days
  - Reduces anatomical dead space
  - Aids weaning from ventilation
- Upper airway obstruction
  - Foreign body
  - Tumour
- Prolonged absence of laryngeal reflexes or ability to swallow
- Airway access

Many tracheostomies are temporary and patients will be able to be weaned from them. Your hospital should have specific guidance on this process. In some situations (e.g. when the patient is unable to protect their own airway) a permanent tracheostomy may be required.

In the case of a mini-tracheostomy, this is always temporary and can only be used for suctioning/to stimulate a cough.

Types of tracheostomy tube
Figure 13.2 shows different types of tracheostomy tube and Table 13.2 indicates when these tubes may be used.

Essential equipment
This is a general guide to equipment at the bedside of ward-based surgical or percutaneous tracheostomy patients. See your own hospital policy for individual units.
- **Tracheostomy dilators** only to be used by persons trained in their use
- **Spare tracheostomy tubes** (1 same size, 1 a size smaller – same make as tube in place)
- **Trachy tapes**
- **Spare inner cannulae** for cleaning purposes (double-lumen tubes only)
- **Inner tube cleaners and sterile water** – clean with sterile water and never leave inner cannulae to soak
- **Oxygen supply and tracheostomy mask**

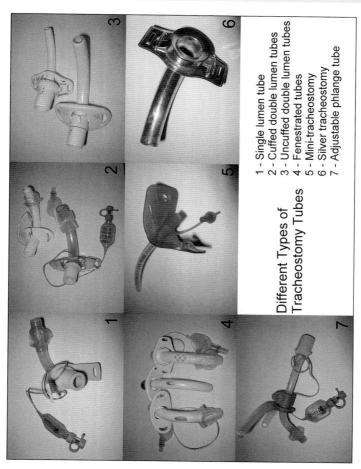

Different Types of
Tracheostomy Tubes

1 - Single lumen tube
2 - Cuffed double lumen tubes
3 - Uncuffed double lumen tubes
4 - Fenestrated tubes
5 - Mini-tracheostomy
6 - Silver tracheostomy
7 - Adjustable phlange tube

Figure 13.2 Tracheostomy tubes.

13

Table 13.2 Tracheostomy tubes

1. Cuffed tube – single lumen	Outer tube only – increased risk of blockage over double-lumen tubes Short-term use (7–10 days) Used for invasive ventilation
2. Cuffed tube – double lumen	Used for invasive ventilation Suitable for long-term use (up to 28 days) Inner tube can be cleaned/replaced
3. Uncuffed tube – double lumen	Used in weaning when not requiring ventilation Patient must be able to swallow oral sections; if not requires cuffed tube
4. Fenestrated tube	Hole/series of holes in the outer tube allows air to pass over the vocal cords allowing speech when speaking valve used or tube is occluded **! Solid inner tube must be inserted for suctioning**
5. Mini-tracheostomy tube	Small tracheostomy tube used only for suctioning Size FG10 suction catheter is largest that can be used Small spigot has to be opened to suction Breathing, swallowing and talking unaffected
6. Silver tube – double lumen	Would be used only if permanent tracheostomy Uncuffed tube
7. Adjustable phlange tube – single lumen	Used when standard tube is too short

- **Appropriate humidification equipment** (e.g. heated or cold water humidification, HME, Buchanon Protector)
- **Suction equipment with appropriately sized catheters** (2 equations can be used to identify appropriate catheter size – check which is used in your hospital. Either: tube size $\times 2 - 2$ or tube size $\times 3 / 2$)
- **Gloves and eye protection**
- **Bowl and sterile water** for flushing suction tubing
- **Ambu bag** or equivalent with tracheostomy connection
- **Clinical waste bag.**

For mini-tracheostomy patient only:
- **Oxygen supply via face mask** – patient will be mouth/nose breathing, therefore use normal mask
- **Suction equipment** – maximum size: FG10 catheters.

Common tracheostomy problems

Thick or plugging secretions

- Check humidification equipment is working and is appropriate for patient.
- Check patient is systemically well hydrated.
- Check if inner cannula needs cleaning/changing.
- Consider obtaining sputum specimen if suspect new infection.

Excessive secretions

- Assess cause
  - New infection (treat as appropriate)
  - Aspiration of saliva – check cuff is inflated
  - Pulmonary oedema – discuss with medical team.

Persistent cough

- Assess cause
  - Tube irritation – aggravated by movement of tube, but may only be minimal secretions present – discuss with MDT
  - Aspiration of saliva – check cuff is inflated
- Some patients require suction kept to a minimum.

Food aspirated on suction

- Swallowing may be impaired by presence of tube
  - Inflate cuff in cuffed tube
  - Strictly enforce NBM if no cuff on tube
  - Treat as aspiration
  - Refer to speech and language therapist ASAP.

Haemoptysis

> Be Aware!
>
> A <u>small</u> amount of blood on suction is common immediately post tube insertion or after head/neck surgery and is not of concern. In all other situations report any blood on suction to MDT.

Consider:

- Is suction pressure less than 20 kPa?
- Has suction catheter hit carina?
- Has suction only been applied when catheter is withdrawn?
- Has suction taken place with a fenestrated inner tube in place?
- Is patient's clotting abnormal?

Unable to access for suction

Consider:

● Is catheter correct size?
● Is tube blocked? – see emergency situations below
● Does the tube position look correct? – see emergency situations below.

Emergency situations

There are three emergency situations with a tracheostomy tube:

● Blockage
● Displacement
● Haemorrhage.

In each situation, prompt responses will improve outcome for the patient.

In all situations pull the emergency alarm to ensure you get help quickly!
If there is bleeding leave the tracheostomy tube in and summon help
immediately.
If initial action to remedy a blocked or displaced tracheostomy tube fails,
the airway is compromised. CALL FOR HELP IMMEDIATELY AND DEFLATE
THE CUFF. **If in doubt, pull the tube out** and manage the airway from the
top. See your local policy for details.

Totally or imminently blocked tracheostomy tube

Thick secretions or a blood clot can potentially block the tube (Table 13.3).

Displaced tracheostomy tube

● Causes
    ● Patient pulling at the tube
    ● An explosive cough when the ties are not tight enough resulting in the
      tube sitting in the pre-tracheal space.
● NB: The patient may show similar signs to a blocked tube or may not be
  distressed at all. A timely assessment is key (Table 13.4).

Haemorrhage

● A major bleed is a very rare complication. Speed of action is very important
  in this instance.
● Bleeding may be:
    ● Early – shortly after insertion
    ● Late – after the tube has been present for a period of time (Table 13.5).

Table 13.3 Blocked tracheostomy tube

Signs of blockage (or imminent blockage)	Increased work of breathing/use of accessories Decreased saturations Cyanosis Audible harsh breath sounds/or absent if having extreme difficulty
Treatment	**GET HELP IMMEDIATELY** Provide oxygen – maximum flow rate (If double lumen) Remove inner cannula and replace with a clean one. This may be enough to clear the blockage Deflate cuff if present (this may allow some air flow around tube) Suction down tracheostomy tube **If unsuccessful, or you feel the patient is having extreme difficulty, remove tube by:** ● deflating cuff ● undoing ties ● removing tube in a down and out motion Provide airway assistance from the top using Ambu bag and mask This is the reason you must always call for help first!

Table 13.4 Tracheostomy tube displacement

Signs of displacement	Increased work of breathing Tube sitting at a strange angle (in this situation the patient may not be in any distress) Surgical emphysema Decreased saturations Cyanosis Unable to pass suction catheter
Treatment	**GET HELP IMMEDIATELY** Can patient breathe? **YES** – apply facial oxygen **NO** – remove the tube and manage the airway from the top To remove tube: ● deflate cuff ● undo ties ● remove tube in a down and out motion Provide airway assistance from the top using Ambu bag and mask This is the reason you must always call for help first! NEVER TRY TO RESITE/REPLACE A TUBE UNLESS YOU ARE SPECIFICALLY TRAINED TO DO SO. IT IS HIGHLY LIKELY TO GO STRAIGHT BACK INTO THE PRE-TRACHEAL SPACE AND YOU WILL HAVE LOST VALUABLE TIME

13

Table 13.5 Haemorrhage

Signs of haemorrhage	Blood oozing from around tracheostomy – this may be a trickle or a pulsing flow
Treatment	**GET HELP IMMEDIATELY** Provide oxygen – maximum flow rate Hyperinflate cuff (this pressure may staunch a big bleed) Suction to clear any blood from airway NEVER REMOVE THE TUBE IN THIS INSTANCE. YOU WILL NEED THE SKILLS OF THE CRASH TEAM FOR THIS TYPE OF PATIENT!

Further reading

Hough A (2001) Physiotherapy for people undergoing surgery. In: Physiotherapy in respiratory care, 3rd edn. Cheltenham: Nelson Thornes.

National Institute for Health and Clinical Excellence (2007) Acutely ill patients in hospital. Clinical guideline 50. London: NICE.

Ridley SC, Heinl-Green A (2002) Surgery for adults. In: Pryor JA, Prasad SA (eds) Physiotherapy for respiratory and cardiac problems, 3rd edn. Edinburgh: Churchill Livingstone.

Singer M, Webb AR (2005) Oxford handbook of critical care, 2nd edn. Oxford: Oxford University Press.

CHAPTER 14

Calls to the neurological/neurosurgical unit

Lorraine Clapham

This chapter covers:
- Key points to consider in the management of the neurological patient
- The brain-injured patient
- The spine-injured patient
- The neuromedical patient.

INTRODUCTION

Disease or injury to the nervous system may affect the rate, pattern and depth of ventilation. Swallow, cough and clearance of secretions may also be affected, and will increase the risk of aspiration pneumonia. On admission to hospital, arterial blood gases may be normal, but respiratory function can deteriorate very quickly, leading to respiratory failure. The physiotherapist needs to be vigilant in the monitoring of these patients. It is important to try to prevent problems and identify and act upon any deterioration as quickly as possible.

> **Remember**
> It is usually reduced ventilation and poor airway protection rather than primary lung pathology that causes respiratory failure in these patients.

KEY POINTS TO CONSIDER IN THE MANAGEMENT OF THE NEUROLOGICAL PATIENT

Respiratory management of the neurological patient depends upon:
- Airway protection, i.e. maintaining a patent airway
- Adequate ventilation.

Features of a patent airway
- Quiet relaxed breathing
- Effective cough capable of clearing secretions
- Safe swallow, i.e. no evidence of aspiration (e.g. cough with food/drink).

Table 14.1 Inadequate ventilation

Features of inadequate ventilation	Result
● Altered respiratory drive ● Alveolar hypoventilation ● Sputum retention ● Aspiration ● Respiratory muscle fatigue	● $\downarrow O_2$ ● $\uparrow CO_2$ ● Respiratory failure type II, i.e. $\uparrow CO_2$ & $\downarrow O_2$ ● Ventilatory failure

If the patient is unable to protect their airway, airway protection techniques will need to be considered.

Airway protection techniques
● Positioning: on side or recovery position
● Manual: chin lift, jaw thrust
● Mechanical: oral/nasal airways, cuffed tracheostomy/endotracheal tubes.
Table 14.1 shows the features of inadequate ventilation.

> **Hazard**
> Cerebral oxygenation and oxygenation to other parts of the body are provided by a patent airway.
> **Occlusion of the airway will result in death.**

NEUROLOGICAL CONDITIONS

Patients tend to fall into one of three main disease categories:
● Brain injury (including surgery)
● Spinal cord injury
● Peripheral neuropathies and neuromuscular disorders.
Respiratory problems encountered within the same disease category are often similar. However, some groups of patients within a category are considered to be 'high risk', i.e. clinically less stable, and therefore have more precautions and contra-indications associated with their treatment. Common respiratory problems will be considered first followed by an example of the management of a 'high-risk' patient from each category.

Brain-injured patient
● Head injury
● Cerebral bleed

- Cerebral infection
- Tumour.

Damage to the brain at the time of injury is irreversible. The aim of treatment is to prevent a secondary cerebral insult leading to further damage, i.e. cerebral ischaemia.

Causes of secondary damage
- Hypoxaemia – $\downarrow O_2$
- Hypercapnia – $\uparrow CO_2$
- Hypotension – $\downarrow BP$
- Reduced cerebral perfusion pressure (CPP)
- Raised intracranial pressure (ICP).

Aim of treatment
- Airway protection
- Normal gaseous exchange
- PaO_2 kept above 12 kPa
- $PaCO_2$ normal to low values (4.0–4.5 kPa) if patient is ventilated
- Maintenance of CPP pressure above 70 mmHg
- ICP below 20 mmHg.

Aim of physiotherapy
To maintain or improve gaseous exchange without compromising CPP, which would lead to cerebral ischaemia.

Normal values
- ICP = intracranial pressure (0–10 mmHg)
- MAP = mean arterial pressure (60–70 mmHg)
- CPP = cerebral perfusion pressure (60–70 mmHg)

e.g. MAP (70) – ICP (10) = CPP (60).

Table 14.2 shows common problems in the neurological patient and Table 14.3 shows common issues in the neurological patient.

HEAD-INJURED PATIENT: CALL OUT
Common problems
- Aspiration pneumonia
- Lobar collapse.

Table 14.2 Common problems in the neurological patient

Common problems	Treatment modification
● Reduced conscious level	● Close 24 h monitoring. Work with nursing colleagues to identify problems and implement treatment plan as appropriate
● Unable to protect airway	● Use airway protection techniques
● Aspiration pneumonia	● Is the patient safe to continue with eating and drinking? Request speech and language therapy referral
● Sputum retention	● Suction ● Postural drainage ● Chest vibrations/shaking
● Hypoventilation, atelectasis	● Manual hyperinflation ● IPPB, NIV ● **(See precautions for the above)**
● Type II respiratory failure i.e. $\uparrow CO_2$ $\downarrow O_2$	● Will need anaesthetic opinion, as ventilation may be required

Questions to ask on the telephone

You need to ask:

- Reason for call out, e.g. aspiration?
- Any other injuries?
- Self-ventilating/ventilated?
- Can they protect their airway?
- Result of ABGs, chest X-ray?
- How stable are they? – cardiovascular, intracranial, i.e. CPP, ICP
- Have parameters been set? – e.g. CPP must be maintained at?
- Precautions/contraindications to treatment, e.g. fracture of base of skull (**BOS**).

Questions to ask the ward staff

You need to ask:

- What is the patient's response to handling/procedures?
- Does **ICP** rise? **CPP** fall? How much? How long does the ICP/CPP take to settle? Hopefully almost immediately. If not, risks of treatment will need to be considered and discussed with the team.

Table 14.3 Common issues in the neurological patient

Common issues	Advice
● High ICP (NB: This may be due to respiratory problem, e.g. $\downarrow O_2$, $\uparrow CO_2$ due to sputum retention and therefore need physiotherapy treatment) ● Unstable haemodynamics (may be exacerbated by sedation, therefore need to increase CVS support) ● Low CPP. If ICP is raised and blood pressure falls CPP will fall which will cause cerebral ischaemia ● Need to modify techniques to minimize effect on ICP, BP and CPP	● Constantly monitor effects of your intervention ● Keep treatment time short ● Ensure that respiratory therapy is indicated, e.g. sputum retention. Pulmonary oedema is not an indication for treatment ● Nursed at 15–35° to reduce ICP (only if they have a protected airway) ● Head kept in midline to avoid decreased venous return from the head due to obstruction of neck veins, which will $\uparrow$ICP ● When changing patient's position, do so slowly ● Tapes securing endotracheal tubes, cervical collars, should not be too tight ● Talk to and reassure patient. Explain what you are doing
● NB: The ventilated patient	● Ensure adequate levels of sedation before start of treatment
● NB: Patient with a cerebral bleed, i.e. subarachnoid haemorrhage	● Risk of further bleed, therefore avoid coughing (can be substituted with ACBT and huffing) ● Caution with activities that affect CVS stability

Information from the charts and monitors

● Note observations and any pattern to changes.
● Note if changes relate to changes in patient's position – you may need to avoid these positions.

Your respiratory assessment

Establish if treatment is required, e.g.:

● Sputum retention
● Lobar collapse.

Consider risks:

● If ICP ≤15 with CPP 70 and stable = low risk
● If ICP 15–20 and CPP 70, settles quickly after treatment within 5 minutes = moderate risk
● If ICP >20 and CPP low = high risk

14

What do you do if the patient is in the moderate- to high-risk group but is severely hypoxic?

You must be confident that you can improve gaseous exchange by removal of secretions and/or reinflation of collapsed areas. Risk associated with treatment must be minimized. Optimize the situation and proceed with great care. If you are unsure discuss the case with the medical team.

Treatment precautions

- Manual hyperinflation – low volumes/rate will increase CO_2 and increase ICP. Cardiac output may fall and cause a fall in MAP and CPP – adapt the breath size and speed accordingly.
- Chest vibrations – smooth and gentle – check effect on ICP and CPP.
- Postural drainage – if ICP in normal range and stable, patient may tolerate horizontal position; if not, head-up position will be required.

Treatment contraindications

- Head-down position – this will increase ICP.
- Nasal airway, nasal suction, NIV, CPAP via a face mask is not permitted for patients with facial or skull base fractures or surgery that involves a transnasal approach, e.g. pituitary tumours.

Monitors and equipment

- Intracranial pressure monitor – records ICP
- Ventricular drain – permits drainage of cerebrospinal fluid
- Cerebral function monitoring – CFM
- Jugular bulb oxygen saturation – indicates cerebral blood flow in relation to cerebral oxygen demand (range 50–75%).

Surgical procedures

This may involve drilling, cutting or removing bone, e.g.:

- Burr hole
- Craniotomy
- Craniectomy.

Inserting drains, e.g.:

- Wound drains
- CSF drainage, e.g. ventricular drain.

> **Remember**
>
> The postoperative management of patients may vary in different neurological units, e.g. to clamp or not clamp ventricular drains when moving a patient. Each procedure will have its own associated precautions and contraindications. You are not expected to know everything. It is essential that you liaise with the staff who are directly involved in the patient's care. They will be able to advise you on what is their unit's current practice. When in doubt discuss with a colleague.

SPINE-INJURED PATIENT

Respiratory function in the spine-injured patient is dependent upon the level of the lesion. Patients with a complete cervical cord injury lose intercostal and abdominal muscle activity and rely on the diaphragm for respiration.

Ascending cord oedema (24–48 h post injury) may result in complete paralysis of the diaphragm (Tables 14.4–14.6).

CERVICAL SPINE INJURY: CALL OUT
Questions to ask on the telephone

You need to ask about the following:

- The injury – stable or unstable?
- Can the patient be moved?
- Any other injuries?
- Result and time of ABGs?
- Chest X-ray?
- Vital capacity – this is a good indication of respiratory muscle strength (normal = 3.5–6 litres or 90 ml per kg of body weight)
- Cardiovascular instability – hypotension, episodes of bradycardia?

Table 14.4 Respiratory function is dependent upon the level of lesion

Level of lesion	Respiratory function
C2	● No respiratory effort
C4	● Partial diaphragm and neck muscles
C6	● Diaphragm and neck muscles
T4	● Diaphragm, some intercostals and neck muscles
T10	● Diaphragm, intercostals, neck and upper abdominal muscles
T12	● Diaphragm, intercostals, neck and abdominal muscles

Table 14.5 Common problems in the spine-injured patient

Common problems	Treatment modifications
● Fear	● Reassure patient
● Reduced inspiratory/expiratory effort ● Atelectasis ● Reduced lung compliance ● Increased work of breathing	● Positioning – supine may be easier for the tetraplegic patient. IPPB, NIV
● Sputum retention/weak cough	● Change of position will aid drainage of secretions. IPPB, NIV. Assisted cough, suction
● Respiratory muscles fatigue ● Hypoxia, hypercapnia	● Keep treatment times short. IPPB, NIV may help. Patient may benefit from use of NIV overnight so that they can rest
● Type II respiratory failure	● You will need anaesthetic advice for further management

Table 14.6 Common issues in the spine-injured patient

Common issues	Advice
Injuries above T6 are associated with haemodynamic instability due to loss of sympathetic outflow, resulting in hypotension and bradycardia	● Care with suction procedures – may cause bradycardia and arrest. Availability of i.v. atropine is recommended. Check that the patient has not been fluid overloaded due to overtreatment of hypotension
CPAP	● May increase O_2 but will not resolve underventilation and CO_2 retention. Use IPPB or NIV

Questions to ask on the ward

Check again with medical staff:

● Level of the injury?
● Stability of the injury?
● Permission to move the patient?

Information from the charts

- Note changes in observations, e.g. vital capacity
- Respiratory rate
- Assess if deterioration was related to change in position
- Haemodynamic stability
- Fluid balance (in an attempt to treat hypotension the patient may have been given large volumes of intravenous fluid resulting in the development of pulmonary oedema).

Your assessment

- Baseline respiratory assessment
- Note respiratory effort
- Breathing pattern
- Respiratory muscles being used
- Effectiveness of cough, able to clear secretions
- Repeat vital capacity measurement.

Treatment precautions

- Assisted cough, manual techniques – should not be attempted without prior training. Must maintain stability of the spine.
- Suction – may cause cardiac arrhythmia – need access to i.v. atropine.
- Positive pressure via a face mask may cause abdominal distension.

Treatment contraindications

- Assisted cough – paralytic ileus, abdominal distension, abdominal injuries.

NEUROMEDICAL PATIENT

Peripheral neuropathies and neuromuscular disorders, e.g.:

- Guillain–Barré syndrome
- Myasthenia gravis.

Early respiratory failure due to neuromuscular paralysis is deceptive. It needs prompt recognition and action. The degree of muscle weakness may not be uniform; there is no correlation between limb power and respiratory muscle power. Patients decompensate rapidly leading to ventilatory failure and respiratory arrest. Anxiety and fear are common. See Tables 14.7 and 14.8 for common problems and issues in the neuromedical patient.

Table 14.7 Common problems in the neuromedical patient

Common problems	Treatment modifications
● Fear	● Reassure patient
● Breathless, increased respiratory rate	● Position to reduce the work of breathing ● Do not lay flat – pressure of abdominal contents against a weak diaphragm can cause respiratory arrest

● Reduced tidal volume
● Low vital capacity
● Reduced lung compliance
● Hypoxia
  – Respiratory muscle fatigue
  – CO_2 retention
	● NIV, IPPB

● Weak cough ● Sputum retention	● Chest vibrations ● Increased tidal volume (IPPB, NIV) ● Assisted cough ● Ensure adequate humidification ● Suction
● Autonomic disturbance ● Hypotension, tachy/bradycardia, e.g. Guillain–Barré syndrome	● Care with suction (ensure availability of i.v. atropine)
● Agitation/confusion/unable to cooperate	● Seek anaesthetic opinion before this stage is reached
● Respiratory failure ● Respiratory arrest	● Ventilation will be required

14

Table 14.8 Common issues in the neuromedical patient

Common Issues	Advice
● Patients decompensate rapidly	● Need constant respiratory monitoring: O_2, respiratory rate, vital capacity 4 hourly, and ABGs if any signs of increasing respiratory distress ● Aim to resolve acute episode, and try to prevent recurrence of respiratory problem ● Have a **current** treatment and **preventive** action plan

Guillain–Barré syndrome: call out

Common problems:

- Hypoxic
- Tired!
- Retaining secretions.

What do you need to ask?

- Did anything precipitate problem, e.g. lying flat to use bedpan?
- What are the ABGs and vital capacity?
- What position was the patient in when tested?

On the ward

- Check with staff when deterioration was noted, e.g. after being given a drink? Aspiration?

From the charts

- Any pattern to deterioration, e.g. reduction in motor power?
- Decline in vital capacity.

Your assessment

- Baseline respiratory assessment
- Note position of patient
- Use of accessory muscles
- Paradoxical chest movement – chest wall moves out, abdominal wall moves in = **weak diaphragm**
- Quality of voice – nasal, wet, gurgle = pharyngeal weakness and risk of aspiration
- Quality of cough – is it effective?
- Vital capacity – 1000 ml or below, patient will need to be considered for ventilatory support.

Contraindications

- Do not lay patient flat.

Precautions

- Suction – cardiovascular disturbance, e.g. bradycardia
- Positive pressure via face mask may cause gastric distension.

Remember

If respiratory function continues to deteriorate due to the progressive nature of the neuropathy, ventilation may be unavoidable.

Further reading

Grundy D, Swain A (2002) ABC of spinal cord injury, 4th edn. London: BMJ.

Harrison P (2000) Systemic effects of spinal cord injury: respiratory system. In: HDU/ICU. Managing spinal injury: critical care, Ch 12. London: Spinal Injuries Association.

Hough A (2001) Disorders in intensive care. In: Hough A (ed.) Physiotherapy in respiratory care: an evidence-based approach to respiratory and cardiac management, Ch 15, 3rd edn. Cheltenham: Stanley Thornes.

Lindsay KW, Bone I, Callander R (1997) Neurology and Neurosurgery Illustrated, 3rd edn. New York: Churchill Livingstone.

CHAPTER 15

Calls to the cardiothoracic unit

Angela Kell

This chapter will cover:
- Cardiac surgery
- Thoracic surgery
- Cardiothoracic trauma
- Cardiology.

CARDIAC SURGERY

This section will detail the postoperative medical management of cardiac patients, the common postoperative problems and physiotherapy management.

Special considerations for assessing cardiac surgery patients

CVS
- Is the patient being paced? If so, are they dependent on it?
- What is the patient's heart rate/rhythm? Is it compromising their blood pressure? What effect is your treatment likely to have on this?
- Inotropic reserve – is there scope to increase pharmacological support if necessary?
- Does BP need to be kept below a certain value to limit risk of graft/conduit leak?

CNS
- Is analgesia sufficient for full assessment and treatment?
- Is there any neurological deficit evident? If so, is swallow/cough reflex affected?
- Is the patient very stiff in the thorax due to anxiety/immobility?

Biochemistry
- Is any concern over perioperative MI?
- What might be affecting fluid balance?
- Is there anything to suggest a postoperative chest infection?

Renal
● Has there been a perioperative renal insult? Is this compromising the respiratory system?

RS
● Are there chest drains in situ? What are they there for?
● Is the respiratory pattern limited by pain or thoracic stiffness?
● Is there any evidence of pneumothorax after chest drain removal? Check the CXR.

Mobilization
● Is there anything to stop you? If so, can it be overcome?
● Consider:
    ● Drips/drains/lines
    ● CVS stability/reserve
    ● Respiratory reserve
    ● Contraindications – PA catheter, IAPB, unstable CVS.

Procedure
Cardiac surgery is normally performed via a median sternotomy, although it can also be done via a thoracotomy incision. The procedure usually requires cardio-pulmonary bypass; however, many surgeons are now opting for 'off pump' surgery for some of their coronary artery bypass grafting (CABG). There is evidence to show that off-pump surgery reduces the incidence of some postoperative complications. Types of surgery include CABG, valve replacement or repair, aortic dissection or aneurysm repair or ventricular remodelling.

Postoperative medical/surgical management
Intra-aortic balloon pump (IABP)
The intra-aortic balloon pump can increase cardiac output by as much as 40%, and will be inserted intraoperatively for patients who cannot maintain adequate blood pressure when they come off bypass. The IABP reduces myocardial workload and improves coronary artery blood flow. Patients with an IABP in situ will be on strict bedrest, and must not flex the hip to more than 30° to avoid displacing it. Positioning of the patient should take account of these restrictions. Manual techniques and bagging may be restricted – follow local guidelines as appropriate.

Pacing
Intraoperatively pacing wires are placed on the myocardium with leads externally connected to a pacing box, as patients are very prone to arrhythmias and intrinsic

pacing problems. See Chapter 3 (page 23) for more details of arrhythmias and ECG interpretation.

Chest drains

Postoperatively, chest drains are routinely positioned in the mediastinum and one or both pleural cavities to drain any residual fluid. Chest drain removal usually occurs when fluid drainage ceases and when there is no visible air leak on coughing. A chest X-ray post drain removal is usually done to ensure there is no pneumothorax. No positive pressure breathing devices should be used until the X-ray is checked. Patients can still be mobilized with a chest drain in situ, although care must be taken to ensure the drainage bottle remains below the site of insertion.

Pharmacological support

The most commonly used drugs for postoperative cardiac patients are summarized in Appendix 4.

Common complications post cardiac surgery are detailed in Table 15.1.

Physiotherapy management

There is no evidence to support prophylactic respiratory physiotherapy for a cardiac surgical population. All postoperative patients should follow a progressive mobilization programme to expedite recovery. If respiratory compromise is identified it should be treated according to cause (Table 15.2). Routine deep breathing exercises are not indicated for patients without respiratory compromise who are able to mobilize.

THORACIC SURGERY

This section will detail the common postoperative problems and physiotherapy management of thoracic patients.

Special considerations for assessing thoracic patients
General
- Exactly where is the incision?
- What is the histology result? Does the patient know this?

CVS
- Is CVS compromised by epidural?

CNS
- Has epidural affected lower limb function?
- Is pain optimized for assessment/treatment?

15

Table 15.1 Common complications post cardiac surgery

Problem	Cause	Medical management	Physiotherapy considerations
Neurological deficit	Intraoperative hypoxia Cerebral ischaemia	May require prolonged ventilation depending on severity; check and manage coagulation	Increased risk of aspiration and respiratory compromise. Advise nursing staff regarding positioning
Pain	Operative procedure, incision site and chest drains Exacerbated by repeated coughing	Analgesia Positioning	Often heightens with anxiety Upper limb movement and thoracic expansion can help ease musculoskeletal stiffness
Renal impairment	Renal hypoperfusion perioperatively	Fluid management, diuresis and ultimately haemofiltration	Haemofiltration lines may limit practicality of mobilization and because of associated hypotension
Hypotension	Cardiac failure Hypovolaemia	Inotropic support, fluid resuscitation, IABP	May limit many physiotherapy techniques including CPAP, IPPB, MHI and mobilization
Hypertension	Pain and agitation Disruption to patient's normal drug regimen	Nitrates for acute episode, recommencing beta-blockers for patients with a history of hypertension	May be aggravated with exercise and inadequate pain control
Arrhythmias	Biochemical derangement (e.g. hypokalaemia), AV bruising intraoperatively, electrical pathway disturbance	Amiodarone, digoxin, pacing, cardioversion	Patient should not be mobilized if rate is fast (> 120) or if blood pressure is compromised – liaise with medical team
Cardiac tamponade	Collection of fluid inside the pericardium which will cause cardiac arrest if not removed	Immediate surgical intervention required	No physiotherapy intervention should be offered

Myocardial infarction	Inadequate myocardial perfusion	GTN infusion, ECG monitoring and troponin level monitoring	Patient should not be mobilized until acute episode has passed – seek medical advice
Sternal wound infection (can lead to mediastinitis)	Infection	Antibiotics, VAC pump	Extrasternal precautions will apply. If sternum fails to unite will alter respiratory mechanics and impede effective cough
Pleural effusion	Premature removal of chest drains, poor positioning of chest drains, low serum protein, poor nutritional status or persistent bleeding	Insertion or repositioning of chest drain. If small will resolve in time and with management of causative factors	Will cause respiratory compromise, but cannot be managed with physiotherapy intervention. Usual chest drain precautions. Optimize oxygen therapy
Pulmonary oedema	Fluid overload or deranged fluid balance	Diuresis. CPAP can be used to increase oxygenation and decrease work of breathing whilst pharmacological management takes effect	Physiotherapy cannot treat pulmonary oedema, although prolonged episodes of pulmonary oedema can lead to infective changes, which may need physiotherapy intervention
Pneumothorax	Failure of pleura to adhere	Chest drain insertion (if small may be conservatively managed)	No positive pressure ventilation should be given to the patient
Lobe collapse	Anaesthetic. Sputum plugging. Pain and insufficient respiratory effort	Oxygen therapy. If ventilated can manipulate settings, e.g. increase PEEP	Requires aggressive management (see Table 15.2)
Chest infection	Sputum retention. Impaired cough	Antibiotics	Optimize analgesia prior to treatment (see Table 15.2). Follow infection control precautions
Hypoxaemia	Impaired gaseous exchange	Depends on cause	Ensure adequate oxygenation throughout treatment

15

Table 15.2 Management of physiotherapy problems

Problem and presentation	Physiotherapy management	Suggested outcome measures
Lower lobe collapse Unilateral or bilateral volume loss on CXR Hypoxaemia Increased work of breathing Poor tidal volume Reduced BS on auscultation Reduced thoracic expansion	Progressive mobilization (if patient has enough reserve): ● Out of bed ● March on spot ● Mobilize on ward ● Use ambulatory oxygen for hypoxaemic patients	Improved breath sounds on auscultation Improved volume on chest X-ray Improved SpO_2 and PaO_2 Reduced respiratory rate
	CPAP: ● Ensure adequate PEEP – larger patients or those with significant collapse will need a PEEP of 10 cmH_2O ● Ensure flow can meet patient's demand – consider size of patient and inspiratory demand (RR) ● If recent drain removal, check X-ray prior to use	
	Bird/IPPB: ● Can be effective if inspiratory flow is reduced due to increased work of breathing ● May have only transient effect – consider use in combination with CPAP ● Ensure flow is high enough to meet demand, then reduce as patient settles ● Pressure should be gradually increased to achieve long, slow, deep breath ● Chest X-ray prior to use	
	Lower thoracic expansion exercises: ● Much less effective than mobilization, but may be only choice if mobilization is contraindicated ● Use in combination with appropriate positioning ● If able, include end inspiratory hold and/or sniff	

Table 15.2 *Continued*

Problem and presentation	Physiotherapy management	Suggested outcome measures
Sputum retention Added sounds on auscultation (crackles, wheezes) Increased work of breathing Increased RR Poor tidal volume Palpable fremitus Wet, weak cough Hypoxaemia Respiratory fatigue	Progressive mobilization (as above) if poor tidal volume is the causative factor	Dry cough No/fewer added sounds on auscultation Improved SpO_2 and PaO_2 Reduced respiratory rate and work of breathing No palpable secretions
	Bird/IPPB: ● Aim to increase tidal volumes ● Intersperse with sputum clearance ● Ensure adequate nebulization ● Use manual techniques in conjunction if able ● Use face mask if patient not able to maintain seal with the mouthpiece or if patient not able to coordinate breathing with the Bird device	
	Manual techniques: ● Must ensure adequate analgesia ● Avoid vibrations/shaking for patients with an unstable sternum	
	Positioning: ● Use in conjunction with above techniques ● Consider CVS status and lines/drains	
	Manual hyperinflation (if intubated): ● If manual techniques alone prove ineffective and if CVS will tolerate ● Aim to increase tidal volumes to mobilize secretions ● Use in conjunction with manual techniques and positioning	
	Suction: ● Endotracheal for intubated patients ● Nasopharyngeal: check clotting is not deranged especially if patient is on haemofiltration and heparinized; use NP airway for repeated suctioning to prevent trauma ● Mini-tracheostomy may be useful in some cases for ongoing sputum retention	
	Supported cough: ● Ensure support (towel, etc.) is clean to prevent wound infection ● Cough-locks can be used ● Reassure patient that sternum is well wired	

15

Respiratory
- Where are the chest drains? What are they doing? Are they on suction?
- What is limiting thoracic expansion? Drains, pain, stiffness, anxiety?
- What restrictions (if any) have been imposed by the surgeon?
- Does the chest X-ray show anything untoward?

Mobilization
- Is there anything to stop you?
- Can the drains come off suction to mobilize?
- What is the most effective alternative?

Procedure

Thoracic surgery is normally for resection of lung tissue to remove a carcinoma (lobectomy, pneumonectomy, wedge resection), management of a recurrent pleural problem (decortication, pleurectomy), removal of bullae (lung volume reduction surgery) or to repair a chest wall deformity. The majority of procedures are carried out via a thoracotomy incision, the extent of which will depend on the nature of the surgery.

Postoperative medical/surgical management

Postoperative monitoring should include heart rate, BP, SpO_2, RR, hourly drain observations and pain scores as a minimum. Common complications after thoracic surgery are given in Table 15.3.

Chest drains

Chest drains are positioned intraoperatively to drain air or fluid from the pleural cavity. The tip of a drain is generally positioned basally for fluid and more apically for air (Figs 15.1 and 15.2). Excellent information on chest drains is available in Pryor and Prasad (2002).

A low-pressure suction tube may be attached to the chest drain to aid drainage. In most instances this suction can be disconnected to facilitate mobilization, the theory being that exercise and thus increased tidal volumes and larger changes in pleural pressures will facilitate drainage. Check your local policy and with ward staff prior to taking a patient off suction.

Chest drain removal for thoracic patients will normally be dictated by local protocols, but is usually performed when fluid drainage ceases and when there is no visible air leak on coughing. A chest X-ray post drain removal is usually done to ensure there is no pneumothorax (see Fig. 15.1).

Table 15.3 Common complications after thoracic surgery

Problem	Cause	Medical management	Physiotherapy considerations
Pain	Incision site Operative procedure and position Chest drain	Analgesia Epidural	Optimize analgesia prior to treatment Check lower limb function prior to mobilization if epidural in situ Upper limb and thoracic exercises in comfortable range can help if exacerbated by anxiety
Persistent air leak in drain	Failure of pleural adhesion	Drains must remain in situ Suction should be applied to drain to facilitate adhesion	Exercise to increase intrathoracic pressure changes can help. Consider exercise bike if on strict suction, otherwise aggressive mobilization including stairs if appropriate
Surgical emphysema	Air leak into subcutaneous space on insertion or removal of chest drain	Oxygen therapy If severe, small superficial skin incisions can be made to release the air	Accurate auscultation around affected area can be difficult
Lung collapse	Sputum plugging, failure of lung to re-expand post intraoperative deflation, pain, insufficient respiratory effort	Depends on cause Analgesia if appropriate If complete lobar collapse due to severe sputum plugging, likely to require bronchoscopy	Requires aggressive physiotherapy management (see Table 15.4)
Sputum retention	Anaesthetic – impaired mucociliary clearance Impaired cough	Prescribe nebulizers where appropriate Ensure adequate hydration	Requires aggressive physiotherapy management (see Table 15.4)
Hypoxaemia	Impaired gas exchange	Depends on cause	Optimize oxygen therapy as part of management and avoid further desaturation
Musculoskeletal dysfunction	Incision site Position on operating table	Analgesia if pain related	May limit thoracic expansion Encourage postural awareness, upper limb movement and follow-up appointment where necessary

15

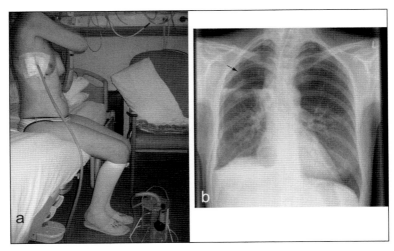

Figure 15.1 Chest drain in situ post-thoracotomy (a) and corresponding CXR (b). Note apical placement of drain (arrow).

Physiotherapy management of acute thoracic patients

Management of the acute respiratory compromised thoracic patient will be dictated by identification of the cause (Table 15.4). This patient group can deteriorate very quickly due to the nature of their surgery. If respiratory compromise is identified they need intensive physiotherapy management immediately. There is little reliable evidence available for physiotherapy management of the thoracic patient and, as for cardiac surgery, no evidence to support the use of prophylactic breathing exercises. Uncomplicated postoperative patients should mobilize on day one postoperatively.

CARDIOTHORACIC TRAUMA

Trauma to the thorax is common in multi-trauma cases, such as RTAs. Isolated thoracic trauma is also common, and potential for complications should not be underestimated.

Rib fractures

Physiotherapy may be indicated for patients with rib fractures if they present with respiratory compromise or sputum retention – manual techniques may be contraindicated depending on site and number of fractures.

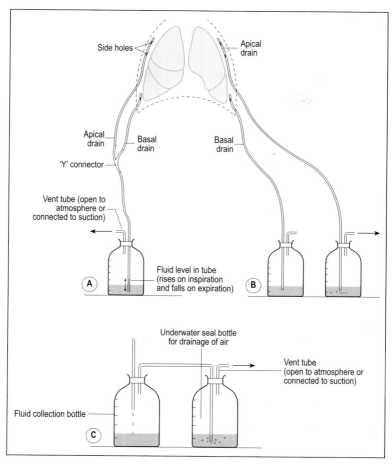

Figure 15.2 Underwater seal chest drainage. (A) Single-bottle system allowing use of one bottle via a 'Y' connector to drain fluid and air. (B) Two separate bottles enabling drainage of air from the apical drain and fluid from the basal drain. (C) Two-compartment drainage system where two bottles are connected in series, the first collecting fluid and the second acting as the underwater seal drainage for air. Reproduced with kind permission from Pryor and Prasad (2002).

Stab injuries

May need surgical repair depending on depth of penetration and entry site.

Lung contusions

Patients often present with very bloody pluggy sputum.

Table 15.4 Management of physiotherapy problems

Problem and presentation	Physiotherapy management	Suggested outcome measures
Lung collapse Reduced BS on auscultation Volume loss on CXR (more than expected with lung resection) Hypoxaemia Increased WOB/RR Reduced thoracic expansion Poor tidal volume Respiratory fatigue	Mobilization ● Can be aggressive if enough respiratory reserve – patient should get SOB to increase TVs ● Monitor hypoxaemic patients closely and use ambulatory oxygen where appropriate ● May be limited to bedside for patients on strict suction ● Consider alternatives (e.g. exercise bike where appropriate)	Improved BS on auscultation Improved volume on CXR Improved SpO_2/PaO_2 Reduced RR/WOB
	LTEEs with end inspiratory hold/sniff ● Less effective than mobilization, but may be only treatment of choice for patients unable to mobilize	
	CPAP ● Only appropriate for some patients with surgeon consent	
	Positioning ● Optimize position in bed if unable to mobilize ● Consider position of comfort if pain is an issue ● Care with drains	

Table 15.4 *Continued*

Problem and presentation	Physiotherapy management	Suggested outcome measures
Sputum retention Added sounds on auscultation Palpable fremitus Wet or weak cough Increased WOB/RR Hypoxaemia Respiratory fatigue	Mobilization (as above) if due to poor tidal volume	Strong/dry cough Reduced added sounds on auscultation Sputum yield Improved oxygenation Reduced WOB/RR Reduced palpable fremitus
	ACBT/LTEEs ● In conjunction with positioning and manual techniques where appropriate	
	Supported cough ● Pillow/towel ● Reassurance regarding wound	
	Positioning ● To increase tidal volume ● To aid postural drainage	
	Manual techniques ● Care over incision site and drain ● May be limited due to pain	
	IPPB ● Must have surgeon consent and guidelines for how much pressure to use ● Not normally appropriate for patients with a persistent air leak ● Monitor drain activity closely (if still in situ) ● Consider positioning and use of manual techniques for optimal effect	

Associated problems

● Pain
● Reduced thoracic expansion and altered breathing pattern
● Impaired cough
● Potential for chest infection/sputum retention
● Hypoxaemia.

Assessment considerations
- Is analgesia sufficient to perform assessment/treatment?
- Are there any other injuries impacting on respiratory status, or which may limit your physiotherapy intervention?
- Is there an associated pneumothorax?
- Is the main problem one which can be helped by physiotherapy intervention?

Treatment considerations
- May need nebulizers to facilitate sputum clearance
- Encourage mobilization
- Care with manual techniques, depending on injuries
- Chest X-ray prior to any positive pressure techniques (possible associated pneumothorax), and obtain consultant consent.

CARDIOLOGY

Acute respiratory physiotherapy is rarely indicated for acute cardiology patients. However this patient group is prone to developing associated problems following a cardiac event, particularly if they are immobile. The most likely scenario will be development of a hospital-acquired pneumonia or infective pulmonary oedema.

Associated problems
- Sputum retention
- Hypoxaemia
- Increased WOB and RR (exacerbated by underlying cardiac pathology)
- Respiratory fatigue and associated weak cough.

Assessment considerations
- What is the medical plan for management of this problem (pharmacological, angioplasty, CABG)?
- What is their cardiac function like? Is this impacting on respiratory status?
- If the patient had chest compressions after an MI are there any rib fractures?
- What does the chest X-ray show – is there evidence of pulmonary oedema?
- Does the sputum look white and frothy? If so, is the main problem pulmonary oedema? This should be managed medically, although CPAP can be indicated in cases of significant hypoxaemia.

Treatment considerations
- Are there any limitations to mobilization (IABP, CVS instability, ECG changes)?

- Ensure adequate oxygenation throughout treatment to prevent further cardiovascular stress.
- Avoid manual techniques if patient has rib fractures.
- How much improvement can you expect if cardiac compromise is also evident?

Acknowledgement

The editors would like to acknowledge the contribution of Sarah Boyce MCSP as author of the Cardiothoracic chapter in the first edition of this text.

Further reading

Brasher P, McClelland K, Denehy L (2003) Does removal of deep breathing exercises from a physiotherapy program including pre-operative education and early mobilisation after cardiac surgery alter patient outcomes? Aust J Physiother 49:165–173.

British National Formulary (2007) London: British Medical Association, Pharmaceutical Press.

Chikwe BG (2006) Cardiothoracic surgery, 1st edn. Oxford: Oxford University Press.

Hulzebos E, Van Meeteren N, De Bie R, Dagnelie P, Helders P (2003) Predication of postoperative pulmonary complications on the basis of preoperative risk factors in patients who had undergone coronary artery bypass graft surgery. Phys Ther 83:8–16.

Jowett N, Thompson D (2003) Comprehensive coronary care, 3rd edn. London: Elsevier Science.

Pasquina P, Tramer M, Walder B (2003) Prophylactic respiratory physiotherapy after cardiac surgery: systematic review. BMJ 327:1379–1385.

Pryor JA, Prasad SA (eds) (2002) Physiotherapy for respiratory and cardiac problems – adults and paediatrics, 3rd edn. Edinburgh: Churchill Livingstone.

15

CHAPTER 16

Calls to the oncology unit

Irelna Kruger and Katharine Malhotra

The purpose of this chapter is to highlight different terminology and specific issues pertinent to the cancer patient.

- Cancer is treated by three main treatment modalities: surgery, radiotherapy and chemotherapy.
- Usually these are used in combination to provide the most effective treatment.
- Treatment depends on the site of the primary cancer, histology and the stage of disease on diagnosis.

As a physiotherapist you will need to be aware that many patients with cancer may have poor performance status prior to treatment due to other co-morbidities. This may increase the risk of respiratory complications and impact upon their ability to comply with physiotherapy intervention.

Patients who are newly diagnosed may have a lack of understanding of their current disease and it is important to be aware how much the patient and relatives/next of kin know about the diagnosis. Many patients may present with high anxiety levels and may have a fear of dying. These factors need to be considered before seeing the patient.

SPECIAL CONSIDERATIONS FOR ASSESSING PATIENTS WITH AN ONCOLOGY DIAGNOSIS

General
- Sudden/gradual change in condition
- Where is the cancer, the primary site +/− evidence of secondary spread
- Stage of treatment, i.e. acute/palliative
- Resuscitation status of patient

- Is the patient limited by pain, fatigue, nutritional status?
- Is the patient in isolation (haematology or neutropenic patients)

CVS
- What are the blood counts and what about anticoagulation? Are they actively bleeding?
- Are they exhibiting signs of sepsis?
- Consider risk of rapid deterioration, especially for haematology patients

CNS
- Are there any signs of altered level of consciousness, possibly brain metastases?
- Is the respiratory drive affected?
- What sedatives/medications is the patient taking?

Respiratory
- Are there any signs of chest disease other than cancer?
- Is there possibility of tumour obstructing the airways?
- Is there possibility of fibrotic or interstitial changes?
- Possible atypical infection (particularly haematology patients)?
- Is there pleural effusion?

Mobilization
- Is there anything to stop you (be aware of possible pathological fractures)?
- Is there the possibility of spinal cord compression? Be aware of local hospital policies regarding manual handling of these patients.

This chapter covers patients presenting with respiratory compromise secondary to:
- bone marrow depression (Table 16.1)
- acute oncology (Table 16.2)
- metastatic oncology (Table 16.3)
- terminal phase of care (Table 16.4).

BONE MARROW DEPRESSION (Table 16.1)

Table 16.1 Bone marrow depression

- Side-effect of chemotherapy
- Increased risk of infection
- More common with leukaemia, myeloma and lymphoma
- Includes neutropenia, thrombocytopenia and anaemia

Common issues	Advice
Neutropenia and neutropenic sepsis	Neutropenia ● A low white cell count ($<0.5 \times 10^9$/L) ● It is difficult to mount a normal response to infection. Patient may present with an unproductive cough and ↑work of breathing ● Use positioning to assist breathing control Neutropenic sepsis ● Temperature above 37.5° ● A low white cell count ($<0.5 \times 10^9$/L)
HAZARD **Thrombocytopenia**	● A low platelet count ($<150 \times 10^9$/L) ● Platelets prevent bleeding and a low count is the commonest cause of bleeding in haemato-oncological conditions ● Patients who are febrile or septic do not maintain platelet levels and require extra support with platelet transfusion ● All hospitals should have a policy for when to transfuse ● Generally, platelets are transfused when levels have dropped to $10–20 \times 10^9$/L ● Physiotherapy intervention should take place during or immediately after platelet transfusion ● Need to know platelet count ● **Need to know if actively bleeding** ● **Minimize intervention if actively bleeding**, i.e. positioning and breathing exercises ● **If requiring suction, ensure count above 20×10^9/L** (check local policy/seek medical advice) ● **Can suction whilst platelets being transfused** ● **Manual techniques**, i.e. percussion and vibrations, can be used to assist with sputum clearance, if no other option to aid clearance. Use a towel to decrease risk of bruising and ensure patient comfort ● **THESE PATIENTS CAN BE TREATED BUT REQUIRE EXTREME CAUTION. IF YOU ARE UNSURE ASK FOR HELP!**

16

Table 16.1 *Continued*

Common issues	Advice
Anaemia	● A low haemoglobin (Hb) count (<13.5 g/dl in men and <11.5 g/dl in women) ● Anaemia occurs in haemato-oncological malignancies due to ↓red cell production and primary disease process itself ● Most centres attempt to keep a patient's Hb level >8 g/dL ● Patients may present with shortness of breath on exertion (SOBOE). Blood is unable to carry sufficient oxygen to the body's muscles, thereby increasing the work of breathing ● *Physiotherapy is not appropriate; medical management should reverse symptoms*

ACUTE ONCOLOGY (Table 16.2)

Table 16.2 Acute oncology

Common issues	Advice
Tumour occluding airway	● Primary lung cancer may cause airway obstruction, atelectasis +/− consolidation behind the tumour, and inflammation around the tumour ● Patient may present with stridor, a harsh wheeze requiring medical intervention ● Patient may sound productive ● **Physiotherapy is not appropriate to clear secretions from behind a tumour** ● Ensure good positioning to ↓work of breathing, O_2 therapy, adequate analgesia and monitor ● Physiotherapy may be appropriate after primary therapy has shrunk tumour
Mucositis	● Inflammation of mucosa of mouth and throat is a common side-effect during and after chemotherapy +/− radiotherapy ● Excessive production of thick, mucoid upper respiratory tract secretions with mouth soreness and ulceration are common ● Patients find it difficult to clear secretions and potentially can be at risk of aspiration ● Mucositis may be mistaken for chest infection ● Advice on breathing exercises and use of high-volume lung clearance techniques to clear upper airway

16

Table 16.2 *Continued*

Common issues	Advice
	● Avoid Yankeur suction if possible at this stage as it may exacerbate symptoms ● Regular saline nebulizers may help to break down secretions making them easier to clear ● Chest infection may co-exist
Aspergillosis	● Opportunistic fungal infection ● Occurs with prolonged neutropenia and with severe bone marrow depression ● Bronchopulmonary aspergilloma can cause cavitating lesions and invade arterioles and small vessels ● Symptoms include malaise, weight loss, fever and productive cough +/− haemoptysis ● If infective sputum present use gentle manual techniques ● **No physiotherapy if frank haemoptysis**
Pneumocystis jiroveci (previously *carinii*) pneumonia (PCP)	● Opportunistic infection in immunocompromised patients causing inflammation of the lungs ● Organisms damage the alveolar lining and produce a foamy exudate ● Symptoms include a dry cough, ↑respiratory rate, breathlessness, hypoxaemia and fever ● Auscultation may often reveal fine, diffuse crackles ● X-ray appearances usually show a haze in the hilar region developing into diffuse symmetrical shadowing (butterfly) ● Medical treatment is with O_2 therapy, respiratory support and antibiotics ● Physiotherapy advice on positioning for relaxation, breathing control and mobilization may be beneficial
HAZARD Pneumonitis	● Inflammatory condition which may be progressive ● Radiation induced, drug related or of viral origin, e.g. cytomegalovirus (CMV), respiratory syncytical virus (RSV) ● Patients present with a dry cough, ↑respiratory rate and breathlessness ● Medical treatment is with high-dose steroids in acute stages ● RSV is treated with nebulized ribavirin (Virazole). **See local policy for administration. HAZARD in pregnancy** ● Physiotherapy advice on positioning for relaxation and breathing control may be beneficial

16

Table 16.2 *Continued*

Common issues	Advice
Disseminated intravascular coagulation (DIC)	● A bleeding disorder with an alteration in the blood clotting mechanism ● Caused by an underlying disease process and is always a secondary condition ● Major causes in the haemato-oncology population are severe sepsis and acute promyelocytic leukaemia ● *Advise caution with physiotherapy intervention due to risk of haemorrhage – therefore, no manual techniques*

METASTATIC ONCOLOGY (Table 16.3)

Table 16.3 Metastatic oncology

Common issues	Advice
HAZARD **Spinal cord compression**	● Caused by primary or metastatic cancer by extradural or intradural compression on spinal cord ● **An oncological emergency → primary treatment with surgery, radiotherapy or occasionally chemotherapy is vital to minimize neurological deterioration** ● May occur at any spinal level and is characterized by motor and sensory loss below level of impairment with bladder and bowel changes ● Patients may experience respiratory difficulties depending on level of compression. Abdominal muscles may also be compromised reducing the patient's ability to cough ● Physiotherapy options will depend on stability of spine, condition of patient and adequate pain control ● **Be aware of your hospital protocols, especially if re-positioning** ● **Check with medics re: stability of spine prior to physiotherapy** (refer to Chapter 14) ● Intervention can include positioning, ACBT, assisted cough and use of IPPB if indicated
HAZARD **Bony metastatic disease**	● Often associated with pain and can lead to pathological fracture and hypercalcaemia ● Common in breast cancer, prostate cancer, lung cancer and myeloma patients ● Usually affects long bones or flat bones of skeleton ● **Important to check for presence of bony disease prior to chest physiotherapy via X-rays/scan reports if available**

Table 16.3 *Continued*

Common issues	Advice
	● **Adequate analgesia** needs to be considered prior to treatment to ensure appropriate positioning ● **Gentle one-handed percussion** may be used if necessary, using a towel for cushioning ● **Use chest vibrations even if rib metastases are present, if no other technique is successful for sputum clearance** ● **Rib fracture may occur – CAUTION** ● Ensure patient feedback for comfort/pain
Hypercalcaemia	● ↑serum calcium levels usually associated with presence of bony metastatic disease ● Symptoms include confusion, lethargy, nausea and vomiting, constipation and thirst ● Physiotherapists need to be aware of this condition as symptoms may compromise effective treatment
Pleural effusion	● Excessive amount of fluid in pleural space ● Symptoms include pallor, cyanosis, dyspnoea, ↑respiratory rate, ↓breath sounds and dullness on the affected side, ↓SpO_2 and chest pain ● Pleural effusion can be readily identified on CXR ● Causes collapse of the surrounding lung tissue ● Medical treatment is by insertion of intrapleural drain ● *Physiotherapy is not appropriate in acute call out situation*
HAZARD **Superior vena cava** **obstruction (SVCO)**	● Primary or metastatic in nature ● Caused by extrinsic or intrinsic compression of superior vena cava ● Usually associated with lung cancer with direct compression from a mass in the right main bronchus, or lymphoma with compression from the mediastinal or paratracheal lymph nodes ● Presents with swelling of neck, upper trunk, upper extremity, dyspnoea with hypoxia, cough and chest pain ● Medical treatment is essential with radiotherapy or chemotherapy ● **Physiotherapy is not appropriate**

16

Table 16.3 *Continued*

Common issues	Advice
Ascites	● Excessive fluid in peritoneal cavity ● Symptoms include abdominal distension and discomfort, nausea and vomiting, leg oedema, and dyspnoea ● Medical treatment is with drug therapy and drainage of peritoneal cavity via a catheter (paracentesis) ● Ascites will compromise diaphragmatic excursion ● Positioning will be difficult ● Forward lean sitting/side lying may be options
Lymphangitis carcinomatosa	● Diffuse infiltration of lymphatics of lungs by cancer cells ● Symptoms include dyspnoea, cough +/− pleuritic chest pain and central cyanosis ● Medical treatment is with drug therapy (corticosteroids and O_2 therapy) ● **Physiotherapy is not appropriate** ● **Advice on positioning may be of some benefit to assist breathing control**

TERMINAL PHASE OF CARE (Table 16.4)

Table 16.4 Terminal stage of disease

Common issues	Advice
Death rattle	● A rattling noise produced by secretions in back of throat oscillating in time with inspiration and expiration ● Can be distressing for relatives, carers and other patients ● Anti-secretory agents are useful, e.g. glycopyrronium or hyoscine ● *Physiotherapy is not appropriate but explanation that patient is not distressed may ease family's anxieties* ● Advice regarding positioning may be beneficial ● Would not encourage use of suction as can increase secretions further
Terminal restlessness	● Common in period immediately preceding death ● Use of sedation may be necessary to keep patient comfortable

● Physiotherapy intervention is limited in these stages
● It can be distressing to feel helpless in these situations but you should be able to recognize your professional limitations
● Support should be sought from peers

16

There are some specific pieces of equipment that are often used in the cancer setting. These include the following.

Hickman catheter
- Used for long-term venous access
- Skin-tunnelled catheter lying in subcutaneous tunnel and exiting midway from anterior chest wall
- Introduced via subclavian vein
- Tip lies in superior vena cava or right atrium.

PICC line
- A long, thin, flexible tube known as a catheter
- Inserted into one of the large veins of the arm near the bend of the elbow
- It is then slid into the vein until the tip sits in a large vein just above the heart
- The PICC line can be used to give treatments such as chemotherapy, antibiotics, intravenous fluids and nutritional support.

Syringe driver
- Portable battery-operated infusion pump
- Used for administration of drugs via a subcutaneous route
- Used for analgesics, anti-emetics, dexamethasone and anxiolytic sedatives
- Often inserted into upper arm or thigh.

Epidural infusion (via an indwelling spinal catheter or intra-thecal catheter)
- Epidural analgesia is administration of analgesics into epidural space
- Used for postoperative pain control or treatment of chronic intractable pain.

KEY POINTS
- Check blood counts!
- Patients often fatigue quickly – keep treatments short
- Consider analgesia and do not forget importance of positioning for patients in pain
- Modify treatments if bony metastatic disease and be aware of presence or risk of spinal cord compression
- Good positioning is essential for breathless patients and those with increased work of breathing – do not rush!
- Unproductive cough: positioning and breathing control are useful. Seek medical advice regarding simple linctus
- Terminal phase of disease: think about comfort – you may not change the pathology

16

Acknowledgement

The editors would like to acknowledge the contribution of Nicola Thompson MCSP as co-author of the Oncology chapter in the first edition of this text.

Further reading

Dougherty L, Lister S (2004) The Royal Marsden Hospital manual of clinical nursing procedures, 6th edn. Oxford: Blackwell Science.

Grundy M (ed.) (2000) Nursing in haematological oncology. London: Baillière Tindall.

Hoffbrand AV, Pettit JE (1999) Essential haematology, 3rd edn. Oxford: Blackwell Science.

Hough A (1996) Physiotherapy in respiratory care, 2nd edn. Cheltenham: Stanley Thornes Publishers.

Otto SE (ed.) (1997) Oncology nursing, 3rd edn. St Louis, MO: Mosby.

Thompson N, Chittenden T (1998) The sepsis syndrome and the cancer patient: respiratory management and active physiotherapy. Eur J Cancer Care 7:99–101.

Tschudin V (1996) Nursing the patient with cancer, 2nd edn. London: Prentice Hall.

Twycross R, Wilcock A (2001) Symptom management in advanced cancer, 3rd edn. Oxford: Radcliffe Medical Press.

16

CHAPTER 17

Calls to the paediatric unit

Paul Ritson

This chapter outlines calls to the paediatric unit; it is sometimes more daunting to be called to a paediatric unit than it is to be called to the paediatric intensive care unit (PICU). The levels of monitoring on the wards are much less than you would find on a PICU, so your observational skills will be vitally important. From the moment the telephone rings, to the time you start treatment, you should gather and analyse information, to formulate an action plan. **DON'T PANIC!**

INAPPROPRIATE CALLS

Unfortunately, your call out may sometimes be inappropriate. Table 17.1 lists conditions that require extreme caution or are totally contraindicated for treatment.

KEY ASSESSMENT NOTES

Before attempting assessment, be aware that gaining consent in paediatrics is different from that in adults. The assessment process is also slightly different (see Chapter 4). When assessing a paediatric patient, it is vitally important to include all body systems as they interact and can affect your assessment and treatment of choice.

Cardiovascular system

Is the patient cardiovascularly stable? (see Appendix 2 for normal values.)

Blood pressure
● Is BP normal for the child's age?

Heart rate
● Is the heart rate normal for the child's age?
● Is the heart rhythm normal?

Neurological system

Could the patient's neurological status affect your treatment?

Table 17.1 Conditions requiring caution and contraindications

Condition	Explanation	Physiotherapy role
Stridor	Harsh sound heard on inspiration. Caused by swelling/oedema/obstruction in upper airway. Usual treatment includes humidification, adrenaline (epinephrine) nebulizers or intubation/tracheostomy	**Do not touch!**
Croup	Viral inflammation of upper respiratory tract. Characterized by a barking cough	**Do not touch** unless airway protected by an **endotracheal tube**
Bronchiolitis	Inflammation of the bronchioles. Mainly seen in winter	**! Physiotherapy will cause hypoxia** Treat only superimposed chest infection/lobar collapse
Whooping cough (pertussis)	Upper respiratory tract swelling. Paroxysmal cough and vomiting. Apnoeas common. May require ventilation	! Physiotherapy may make the patient worse
Acute epiglottitis	Swollen epiglottis. Airway blocks quickly. Child should be sat upright	**Do not touch!**
Acute pneumonia	Consolidation phase. Non-productive and painful	**Position for ventilation/perfusion matching**
Bronchospasm	Constriction of the airways caused by spasm of the bronchial muscles	! Treat cause of bronchospasm and reassess patient
Inhaled foreign bodies	Common in children	**Do not be persuaded to treat!** Bronchoscopic removal first, then physiotherapy if indicated
Undrained pneumothorax	Could cause tension pneumothorax	**Do not use IPPB/CPAP** Position for ventilation/perfusion until chest drain inserted and give oxygen
Severe CVS instability	Unacceptable blood pressure or heart rate for age of patient	**Physiotherapy contraindicated** **Use of IPPB/CPAP contraindicated**
Uncontrolled seizures	Hypoxia and aspiration may occur	Reassess when seizure activity reduces
Pulmonary embolus/clotting disorders	Patient may bleed or throw off clots if treated	! If unsure, discuss with senior staff

17

Temperature
- Infants can suffer seizures if pyrexial (febrile convulsion).

Intracranial pressure
- Head-injured patients should be monitored closely for abnormal neurological signs, e.g. photophobia, restlessness, headaches, neck stiffness, vomiting.

Pre-existing pathology
- Does the patient have a neurological condition that causes respiratory problems or alters your treatment choice?

Orthopaedic

Does your patient have any orthopaedic problems that could affect your treatment?

Fractures
- Spinal and limb fractures will affect the positioning of your patient.
- Follow your hospital's protocols carefully.

Pre-existing conditions
- Kyphoscoliosis, chest or limb deformities alter the normal mechanics of respiration, predisposing to respiratory disease.
- Positioning may be difficult, but still try to be effective.

Surgery
- Orthopaedic surgery, especially spinal, can alter the mechanics of respiration and will dictate the positions your patient is allowed to be in.
- Follow your hospital's protocols carefully.

Fluid balance
Positive balance
- Expect copious loose secretions and pulmonary oedema.

Negative balance
- Thick viscous secretions leading to mucous plugging and sputum retention.

Drugs
Review the patient's drug charts.

Inotropes
- Cardiovascular support drugs, usually only seen on PICU, e.g. adrenaline (epinephrine), dobutamine, milrinone, noradrenaline (norepinephrine), dopamine.

Painkillers
- Look at the route of administration: i.v., i.m., oral, rectal, epidural.
- Is pain relief adequate? Does it require time to take effect? E.g. morphine, diclofenac, paracetamol, fentanyl.

Sedatives
- Look at route of administration.
- E.g. midazolam, promethazine, chloral hydrate, clonidine.
- Propofol not used in children under 1 year.

Bronchodilators
- Must be given before physiotherapy and before inhaled steroids.
- In infants, current research suggests beta-2 agonists are effective.
- Salbutamol and ipratropium bromide can be nebulized together to treat bronchospasm.

Steroids
- Inhaled or systemic.
- E.g. prednisolone, budesonide (Pulmicort).
- Long-term systemic steroids cause osteoporosis, even in children.

Diuretics
- Can indicate pre-existing cardiac pathology or pulmonary oedema.
- E.g. furosemide (frusemide).

Carry out a full paediatric respiratory assessment, including type of surgery, incision site, relevant past medical history and special postoperative instructions.

AIMS OF PHYSIOTHERAPY TREATMENT
- **Gain patient/carer trust and cooperation**
- Ensure adequate analgesia
- Aid removal of secretions
- Reduce work of breathing (WOB)
- Prevent/treat atelectasis.

CALLS TO THE PAEDIATRIC SURGICAL WARD
See Tables 17.2 and 17.3 for common problems in the paediatric surgical ward and common issues and advice for the paediatric surgical ward, respectively.

Table 17.2 Common problems in the paediatric surgical ward

Common problems	Treatment modifications
Atelectasis	● Good positioning is essential ● Sitting upright is effective for infants who frequently suffer upper lobe collapse – use a car seat to achieve this, making sure the patient is safe and supported ● Alternate side-lying aids re-expansion of the uppermost lung; regular repositioning is vital ● Blowing games or bubble bottles and incentive spirometers are useful in older children ● Mobilize patient if possible. This may involve play, standing at a table to play or other creative ways of encouraging a child to their feet! ● IPPB can be used effectively, usually in children over 6 years of age ● CPAP can be used in any age group (see Chapter 20)
Sputum retention	● Occurs due to pain, immobility or inability to cough for whatever reason ● Ensure adequate analgesia ● Humidify with face mask in children and head box in infants ● 5 ml 0.9% saline nebulizers can be used hourly if prescribed ● If patient unable to cough spontaneously or to command, nasopharyngeal suction may be indicated if secretions are adversely affecting the respiratory status of the child ● Position for comfort and drainage ● Assess the use of the 'head-down' tip position very carefully, as reflux, vomiting and aspiration occur more easily in this position ● The 'head-down' position also splints the diaphragm, reducing respiratory function ● Mobilize patient if possible ● Use cuddly toys for wound support when coughing **(if the toy is clean!)**
Increased work of breathing	● 'Head-up' position reduces load on diaphragm and reduces reflux of gastric contents ● Avoid supine as this is the worst position for gas exchange and increases the risk of aspiration when vomiting ● Alternate side-lying with head up reduces load on diaphragm and improves gas exchange ● Prone-lying is best position for gas exchange and reducing WOB ● **If using prone-lying, patient MUST be closely monitored** by nursing staff and have the following monitors in situ: SpO_2, apnoea mat, and ECG with all alarms enabled and audible

17

Table 17.3 Common issues and advice for the paediatric surgical ward

Issue	Advice
Pain	● An infant in pain usually cries inconsolably ● A child in pain will also cry, but can also be unusually quiet until disturbed ● A child in pain will not cooperate! ● Check timing of analgesia and route of administration – how long will it take to become effective? ● Can supplemental analgesia be given? ● Beware of opiate depression of the CNS ● Cooperative children can use Entonox if prescribed and the clinician is trained to administer it
Poor cooperation	● Very common! See Chapter 4 ● Try trickery; use toys or play ● Distraction by carers/nurses during treatment ● **Never force or hold a child down unless they are in danger**
Poor position	● A child in pain is usually slumped in bed – use supported positioning to improve pain and improve respiratory function ● Children/infants with neurological disorders can have increased extensor tone when in pain. Ensure adequate analgesia and optimize position ● Early mobilization/sit out of bed if possible
Parents	● Will be very anxious ● **Always gain consent for treatment (see Chapter 4)** ● Gain parents/carers' trust and cooperation ● Involve parents/carers in treatment if possible ● Children may be more cooperative if parents/carers are not around at the time of treatment ● Some children may only do treatment with a parent/carer
Oxygen delivery	● Humidification is vital if secretions are thick, or if FiO_2 is over 0.28 (over 2 litres per minute) ● Use a head box or face mask for humidification ● Humidification is poor via nasal cannulae, but may still be used in some centres
Timing of treatment	● Never treat a patient immediately after a feed or meal because of the risk of vomiting and aspiration ● Leave at least 1 hour before treating ● Best time to treat would be immediately prior to a feed/meal

17

Table 17.3 *Continued*

Issue	Advice
Blocked nose	● Can cause increased work of breathing even in the absence of other pathologies ● Unblock nose if possible ● Saline drops may still be used in some centres if prescribed
Other pathologies	● Be aware of the patient with complex multiple needs on the surgical ward ● This type of patient can deteriorate very rapidly

COMMON CONDITIONS SEEN ON PAEDIATRIC SURGICAL WARDS

There are many conditions encountered on the surgical wards. Tables 17.4 and 17.5 provide advice on patient groups and equipment. All conditions should be taken into consideration when carrying out a respiratory assessment. Further reading about conditions is strongly recommended. See Further reading at end of chapter.

Table 17.4 Assessment/treatment advice for common conditions on paediatric surgical wards

Condition	Assessment/treatment hints
Idiopathic scoliosis (postoperative correction)	● Altered respiratory mechanics postoperatively ● Chest drains for at least 1 week ● Pain management important ● Ribs removed during surgery – care with manual techniques ● Log roll only – no rotation ● Incentive spirometry and supported cough very effective
Cerebral palsy (CP)	● Usually postoperative orthopaedic surgery in hip spica ● General surgery for fundoplication and/or gastrostomy ● Pain and sputum retention usually the main problems, exacerbated by poor cough ● Effective positioning is vital for respiratory and neurological reasons
Congenital cardiac disorders	● Take special note of patient's colour and SpO_2 – cyanosis and low SpO_2 can be normal in some cardiac conditions ● Refer to local guidelines for acceptable SpO_2 in cardiac patients and postoperative protocols
Congenital diaphragmatic hernia repair	● Depending on the size and duration of hernia, diaphragm may be weakened and affected lung may be underdeveloped/hypoplastic, predisposing to respiratory insufficiency
Abdominal surgery	● Can cause distension, leading to splinting of diaphragm ● Use high side-lying to aid diaphragm excursion
Thoracic empyema	● Chest drains and pain are common ● Position for ventilation and perfusion matching

17

Table 17.5 Monitors and equipment

Monitor/equipment	Explanation
Patient-controlled analgesia (PCA) or nurse-controlled analgesia (NCA)	● If old enough, child will be able to press for analgesia ● If younger or unable to press, nurse **ONLY** can press for pain relief
Pulse oximeter	● Very commonly used postoperatively ● Make sure the probe is attached to the patient and the signal is strong and regular ● Look at the patient as well as the oximeter; if the SpO_2 is reading 30% and the patient is pink, the oximeter is wrong! ● If child wearing nail varnish, SpO_2 will not be accurate – change probe site to ear lobe or toe
Chest drains	● Never clamp unless lifting above waist height ● In most cases it is acceptable to sit a patient out or mobilize the patient ● **If you are unsure about moving a patient with a chest drain, ask senior staff for advice**

CALLS TO THE PAEDIATRIC MEDICAL WARD

Carry out a full paediatric respiratory assessment, including past medical history and the course of this episode. In this group of patients, pre-existing pathology may be particularly relevant and important (Table 17.6).

Common issues on the paediatric medical ward

Many of the issues encountered on the medical ward are similar to those seen on the surgical ward. Those more commonly encountered on the medical ward are mentioned in Table 17.7.

Common conditions seen on the paediatric medical ward

There are many conditions encountered on the medical wards. Pathologies behind these conditions must be taken into consideration when assessing these children (Table 17.8). Further reading is strongly recommended; see end of chapter.

17

Table 17.6 Common problems on the paediatric medical ward

Common problem	Treatment modifications
Atelectasis (as for surgical patient)	● Effective positioning is vital – always position the affected side uppermost to improve ventilation and sputum clearance ● You may need to increase FiO_2 in the short term to achieve this ● Modify position if the patient continues to desaturate ● Position the affected side down to improve oxygenation with consolidated pneumonia ● Avoid 'head-down' position if patient prone to aspiration/reflux ● IPPB/CPAP can be useful (watch pressures given) ● **Mobilize if possible**
Sputum retention (as for surgical patient)	● Common in children with neurological disorders ● Due to poor cough, altered respiratory mechanics and aspiration ● Nasopharyngeal (NP) suction can be very important in this patient group. The technique can be tricky – ask senior staff for assistance ● **Oropharyngeal (OP) suction should be used with extreme caution** – a gag reflex is commonly stimulated rather than a cough reflex; side-lying is essential ● Positioning in alternate side-lying with head up is effective for sputum clearance and comfort ● Humidification is vital if secretions are thick, or if FiO_2 is over 0.28 (over 2 litres per minute) ● Humidification is poor via nasal cannulae, but may still be used in some centres ● 5 ml 0.9% saline nebulizers can be used hourly if prescribed ● Some patients may have used the cough assist machine before – only use if you or the nursing staff are familiar with it (see Chapter 19)
Increased work of breathing (as for surgical patient)	● Ascertain cause of increased WOB and treat accordingly (e.g. pain, sputum retention, anxiety) ● Effective positioning is vital ● High side-lying and supported sitting are useful ● Treat in quiet area if possible ● Ensure nappy or clothes are not too tight as compressing the abdomen can cause increased WOB

17

Table 17.7 Common issues and advice on the paediatric medical ward

Issue	Advice
Poor position	● Good positioning is essential for effective respiration ● Avoid supine
Inappropriate oxygen delivery	● **Beware the dangers of high-flow dry oxygen** ● Always humidify ● Humidification more effective via head box or face mask
Bronchospasm	● Ascertain cause ● Bronchodilator 30 minutes prior to treatment and reassess ● Give via nebulizer or spacer ● Salbutamol and ipratropium bromide can be nebulized together for severe bronchospasm ● Small amounts of bronchodilator can be made up to a greater volume by adding 0.9% saline
Uncooperative child	● Use play and distraction ● Trickery! ● Enlist help of parents/carers, or ask them to leave if a child is 'acting up' with them around ● **Never force a child**
Child with complex needs	● May be unable to cooperate with treatment ● Treatment usually passive ● Speak to and reassure patient ● **Do not attempt to lift/move a larger child by yourself – ask for help**

Table 17.8 Assessment/treatment advice for common conditions on paediatric medical wards

Condition	Assessment/treatment hints
Cystic fibrosis	● Will have set routine – check notes and ask parents/carers ● See postural drainage, PEP, ACBT, Chapter 19 ● May have routine bronchodilator pretreatment ● DNase sometimes given to liquefy mucus – check your hospital policy as to when it should be given ● Check abdomen – a hard abdomen will splint the diaphragm ● Look at lung function tests and compare to previous results ● Exercise very important ● Often uncooperative! ● Be assertive, but not bossy! ● **Never force or restrain a child unless they are in danger** ● Auscultation is often deceptive – crackles sometimes not heard, even in the presence of retained secretions ● Listen to cough: is it dry, tight or productive?

17

Table 17.8 *Continued*

Condition	Assessment/treatment hints
	• NIV is sometimes used in older CF children as a bridge to transplant or to aid respiratory function during acute episodes • Always discuss with senior staff before removing the patient/NIV interface • Sputum clearance techniques can be used while the patient is on NIV and the mask removed for expectoration only if the patient is severely compromised
Asthma	• Positioning for ventilation, perfusion and comfort in acute phase • Use heated humidification • Ensure bronchospasm under control before attempting treatment • **Beware of quiet lung sounds (overwhelming bronchospasm can cause a silent chest – check your stethoscope), fatigue and increasing CO_2 – will need an urgent anaesthetic review**
Bronchopulmonary dysplasia (BPD)	• May be on home oxygen • Find out the patient's normal FiO_2 • Tendency for bronchospasm • Treat as chronic lung disease
Primary ciliary dyskinesia	• Very rare • Develop sputum retention/chest infection rapidly • Treat chest symptoms as for CF
Immunodeficiency	• Treat chest symptoms as for CF
Neurological conditions	• Aspiration, poor cough and sputum retention common • Ask parent/carer (or child, if able) what chest is like normally – what you see may be normal for the child • Assisted cough with abdominal support is effective with degenerative disorders such as Duchenne muscular dystrophy or spinal muscular atrophy • Gravity-assisted postural drainage positions used with care (risk of reflux and aspiration) • CPAP/IPPB and cough assist device used if indicated • **Suction only if secretions are adversely affecting the respiratory status of the child, or if they are uncomfortable** • Always communicate with the child • Get help to position or turn the child • If patient not protecting airway, or if repeated suction is required, consider use of a nasopharyngeal airway • **NEVER** use an oropharyngeal airway (Geudel) in a conscious patient (risk of vomiting and aspiration)

17

Table 17.8 *Continued*

Condition	Assessment/treatment hints

The dying child	● Very uncommon to be called out in these circumstances
	● Ascertain why the call has been made and what the referrer expects
	● Management may include:
	  − Comfortable positioning (side-lying with 'head up' or long sitting, well supported with pillows)
	  − **Suction only if the child is distressed with secretions and unable to expectorate** − technique should be quick, gentle and effective
	● Talk to the child and parents/carers
	● Ensure dignity is maintained
	● This is a distressing time for all concerned; senior staff will always be available for help, advice and support
	● Discuss with team the need for physiotherapy versus time with the family
	● Always check the resuscitation status of the child (full, limited, or no resuscitation)

KEY POINTS
- Be methodical
- Gather appropriate information
- Consider pre-existing pathologies
- Communicate with the child, parents/carers and the multidisciplinary team
- Never underestimate the power of play
- Be very observant
- Frequent reassessment
- Be aware of the signs of respiratory distress (Table 4.3)
- Be aware of contraindications and cautions for treatments (Table 17.1)

Further reading
Jordan SC, Scott O (1989) Heart disease in paediatrics, 3rd edn. London: Butterworths.
Prasad SA, Hussey J (1995) Paediatric respiratory care: a guide for physiotherapists and health professionals. London: Chapman Hall.
Pryor JA, Prasad SA (2002) Physiotherapy for respiratory and cardiac problems, 3rd edn. Edinburgh: Churchill Livingstone.

CHAPTER 18

Calls to the neonatal unit

Alison Carter

This chapter covers treatment in the neonatal unit including aims of treatment, common problems, conditions and issues, assessment, and risks and contraindications.

TO TREAT OR NOT TO TREAT?

Calls to the neonatal unit are rare now that a balance has been achieved between minimal handling and appropriate and timely repositioning of preterm babies to prevent secretion retention and lobar collapse.

The evidence base for treating this group of infants is lacking and therefore treatments should not be routine but restricted to babies who display respiratory distress through specific lobar collapse or thick tenacious secretions.

Hazard

It is generally accepted that the treatment of this client group should not be undertaken unless the physiotherapist is FULLY trained and competent in the care of neonates.

Often simple instructions regarding position changes and adequate suctioning are sufficient in an unstable baby. A deteriorating respiratory status as a result of lobar collapse or retention of secretions will indicate the need for more active assessment and intervention.

- **Neonate** = a baby born from 37 weeks (term is 40 weeks)
- **Premature baby** = a baby born before 37 weeks.

REASONS FOR RISK IN TREATING THESE INFANTS

- Extreme prematurity and low birth weight result in a high incidence of instability with handling

● Immature CNS and lungs
● Long periods of time needed to recover after minimal interventions
● High risk of secondary sequelae (e.g. cerebral bleeds, abdominal/gut bleeds).

AIMS OF TREATMENT
● To maintain a clear airway
● To assist in the removal of tenacious secretions
● To maintain/improve gaseous exchange without further compromising the already fragile, immature infant
● To assist early extubation
● To help prevent further respiratory collapse.

NORMAL VALUES
Table 18.1 shows normal values for neonates.

EQUIPMENT
● Ventilators vary from unit to unit. Nursing staff are there to guide you.
● Ventilators with flow loops can indicate the need for suction when the loop is interrupted with obstruction from secretions.
● CPAP units vary but their use with prongs or a mask has led to earlier extubations. (Care must be taken to keep the nasal passages clear for CPAP to be fully efficient.)

COMMON PROBLEMS, CONDITIONS AND ISSUES
Common problems in the neonatal unit, common conditions in neonates and term babies, and common issues in the neonatal unit are listed in Tables 18.2–18.4, respectively.

Table 18.1 Normal values

Vital sign	Approximate value
Heart rate	Preterm 100–200 b.p.m. Term 80–150 b.p.m.
Blood pressure	80/45 mmHg Aim to keep systolic above 35–45 mmHg
Respiratory rate	30–45 breaths per minute
Saturations	90–96%

18

Table 18.2 Common problems in the neonatal unit

Common problems	Treatment modifications
Lobar collapse (frequently right upper lobe, due to endotracheal tube being too long)	● Modify positioning ● Ensure regular change of position to prevent further collapse ● May use ½ lying/semi-propped position ● Suction with head to the left ● Record and discuss with nursing staff
Secretion retention (increased viscosity and amount)	● Check humidification is adequate ● Use of saline with treatment ● Think of infection, fluid balance and pulmonary oedema (this will affect the nature of response which is appropriate as secretion type will vary) ● Increase frequency of positioning ● May need increased frequency of suctioning especially if the infant has been turned 8-hourly

Table 18.3 Common conditions in neonates and term babies

Common conditions in neonates	Management hints
Respiratory distress syndrome With increased secretions and/or acute lobar collapse	● Regular change of position ● Active techniques not indicated unless collapse is present and does not resolve with repositioning and suction
Chronic lung disease With multifocal collapse Chronic secretion retention CO_2 retention	● Treatment as indicated ● Regular change of position ● Active techniques with effective suction ● Daily assessment
Term baby: common problems Hypoxic ischaemic encephalopathy Meconium aspiration Tracheo-oesophageal fistula Diaphragmatic hernia	● Limitations to positioning due to stability/operation site ● Frequent repositioning ● Effective suctioning ● Treat collapse
Cardiac anomalies: term and preterm	● Treat only if indicated ● Attempt position change even if only minimal movement is possible ● Good liaison with medical/nursing staff as to individual precautions of different cardiac anomalies

18

Table 18.4 Common issues in the neonatal unit

Common issues	Advice
Routine treatments being undertaken	● Individual treatment plans essential ● Assess and re-assess as picture is constantly changing
Chest sounding clear on auscultation, but copious secretions on suction	● An assessment treatment is wise if clinically indicated to clear secretions from the posterior lung bases ● Place prone at least once in every 24 hours ● Record/discuss with colleagues
Infants at 28–29 weeks or less not tolerating side-lying	● Use ¼ turns from prone and supine ● Lungs not fully developed laterally ● Rib cage very compliant ● ¼ turns are tolerated better
Preferential ventilation	● In the presence of one-sided collapse the infant may not tolerate lying on the fully expanded lung ● May need to increase FiO_2 ● Position change for drainage may only be possible for short periods ● NB: Collapse on the opposite side is sometimes possible if an infant is nursed for long periods in one position ● Record and set a plan
Rapid desaturation with appropriate treatment/handling	● Can be pre-empted by pre-oxygenation ● 15–20% initially ● Use of manual breaths on ventilator if secondary bradycardia
Apnoeas of prematurity	● Common; may happen during treatment ● Stimulate baby to breathe, tap bottom or flick heel ● In extremes, manual breaths or Neopuff
Nursing position maintained for long periods of time	● Modified position changes little and often ● Instability may be due to secretion retention; may respond well to gentle more frequent changes in position
Desaturation and long recovery post physiotherapy	● Perform physiotherapy separately from all cares

18

Table 18.4 Continued

Common issues	Advice
Signs of CO_2 retention, increased oxygen requirement with increased secretions	● Change position, assess need for increased suction and manual chest techniques
Dislike by carers in the use of closed suction circuits	● Safer in oscillated babies and those on nitric oxide ● Maintains pressures and PEEP ● Prevents desaturations ● If this is unsuccessful and clear clinical reasoning is demonstrated, traditional suctioning methods can be used as indicated
Occasional inability to clear secretions with closed suction	● ETT may be small ● ETT may be blocked, partially obstructed or kinked ● Change to open suction

THE CALL OUT TO THE NEONATAL PATIENT: WHAT DO YOU NEED TO ASK?

On the telephone
● Has a chest X-ray been done?
● Blood gases: the trend. Stability of the infant and the mode of ventilation
● Platelets, metabolic state (risk of congenital rickets)
● Length of time since birth, respiratory history (respiratory distress syndrome, chronic lung disease, etc.).

On the ward
● Verbal handover
● How the infant handles with cares/suctioning
● Amounts of oxygen increase needed for this
● Results of CXR.

From charts/monitors
● Gases, oxygenation, HR, BP
● Last series of cares and effects
● Nursed constantly in one position?
● Recent respiratory arrest/desaturations/bradycardias/reintubations and the recorded cause.

18

ASSESSMENT

- For guidance on consent issues please refer to Chapter 4
- Number of days from birth, if <7 then use positioning only if less than 35 weeks' gestation
- General response to handling
- Frequency of suction
- Response to change of position
- Colour, respiratory rate, etc.
- Abdominal distension (modify position)
- Cerebral bleeds?

TREATMENT PRECAUTIONS

Remember
If undertaking active techniques, the infant's head MUST always be fully supported. If in doubt do NOT treat and discuss with the team.

- If the infant has neonatal rickets use positioning only.
- Avoid lying on clear lung for long periods of time with collapse on the other side, due to V/Q mismatch.
- Always make note of acute medical state before embarking on active chest techniques, as the infant may be too unstable to cope with more than just a gentle change of position.

TREATMENT CONTRAINDICATIONS

- Head-down position due to high incidence of reflux; this can cause increased cerebral pressure, increased intra-abdominal pressure in the presence of necrotizing enterocolitis (NEC)
- Very low platelets
- Abdominal distension with NEC
- Pulmonary haemorrhage
- Manual hyperinflation: risk of pneumothorax and barotraumas.

RISKS

Table 18.5 lists the main risks to be considered.

TREATMENT TECHNIQUES

Tables 18.6 and 18.7 highlight the treatment techniques and modifications, and techniques contraindicated in neonates, respectively.

Table 18.5 Consider the risks

Are you trained?	● If **no**, simple advice on positioning and suction
	● Discuss with your on call service manager the next day
	● If **yes**, refer to local guidelines for chest treatment in the preterm infant
	● NB: This includes local suctioning standards
	● Liaise with senior nursing/medical staff
Documentation	● Clear, full recording of assessment, treatment and advice given is essential
	● Leave a clear plan of recommendations for reassessment, changes of positioning and suctioning

Table 18.6 Techniques and modifications

Manual techniques	Neonatal modifications
Assessment	● Always treat with the nurse present to assist with alarms, suctioning, etc.
Positioning/postural drainage	● Head down contraindicated
	● Preferential ventilation of uppermost lung, therefore V/Q mismatch
	● Prone improves oxygenation, drains the posterior lung bases and is commonly the most stable position
	● Prone = decreased reflux, decreased respiratory effort and better quality of sleep
	● Regular position changes within tolerance ensure no region of lung remains dependent for long periods of time
Percussion with Bennett face mask	● Always use appropriately sized mask
	● Follow local guidelines on appropriate pressures for percussion (0.5 mmH$_2$O, in infants under 28 weeks)
	● Only treat in 1–2 positions at a time
	● Use 1–2 minutes of percussion in each position, **stopping** if the infant desaturates or demonstrates poor tolerance
	● Suction when secretions have loosened
	● NB: Small infants only tolerate 2 very short treatments with corresponding suctioning
Vibrations (done with the 'pad' of the distal phalanx)	● Applied finely with 2 or 3 fingers throughout expiration, every 2–3 breaths
	● Used appropriately, 3–5 vibes will clear secretions and these can be felt mobilizing under the fingertips
Suctioning as an adjunct to physiotherapy	● In non-ventilated infants and those on nasal CPAP, clearance of the upper airway with nasopharyngeal suction is essential as infants are preferential nose breathers

18

Table 18.6 *Continued*

Manual techniques	Neonatal modifications
Suctioning via ETT (should comply with local suctioning standard)	● Suction orally in ventilated babies; often secretions come around the tube ● Complete suction in 8–10 seconds ● Pressures 6–8 kPa ● Catheter size only half the internal diameter of the ETT (see Chapter 19 – Treatments) ● Insert catheter to 1 cm past the end of the ETT only ● Use saline, if indicated, in the following amounts: 23–28 weeks 0.2 ml; 28–35 weeks 0.4 ml; term plus 0.5 ml

Table 18.7 Techniques contraindicated in neonates

Technique	Reason
Manual hyperinflation	● This is NOT used in the preterm infant ● Risk of pneumothorax ● Does not utilize collateral ventilation as this is not established ● Rescue/resuscitation only ● Used in term or larger babies with caution ● Most units now use the Neopuff which strictly monitors and controls pressures which can be preset to match ventilator pressures ● Follow local guidelines carefully

SUMMARY

It is imperative that wherever chest physiotherapy is practised, especially if this is shared by the nursing staff, the appropriate protocols, teaching and indeed competency frameworks are in place to allow for accountability for any techniques being undertaken.

This recorded information needs to be backed with full clinical reasoning and, wherever possible, evidence-based protocols.

Assessments and treatments should always be individual and not routine; reassessment for every treatment is best practice as sometimes only one treatment may be necessary.

In conclusion, only treat if trained and if in doubt contact a senior paediatric physiotherapist **and discuss with the medical and nursing staff.**

KEY POINTS

● Only treat a neonatal patient if you are specifically trained in this area of care.

● If the baby is very small and fragile with a poor response to handling maintain a hands-off approach.

● Try to avoid treatment in the first week post birth for the very premature infants (increased risk of cerebral bleed).

● If you are called to a neonatal patient and you are not trained in the physiotherapy management of preterm infants **do not** treat the patient. It is better that the nursing staff continue to manage the patient. Contact a senior member of the medical, nursing or paediatric physiotherapy staff for support.

CHAPTER 19

Respiratory physiotherapy treatments

Alison Draper and Paul Ritson

The following (alphabetical) list of treatment options will assist you in your treatment planning. Each individual patient will respond uniquely; therefore you may consider certain precautions or contraindications appropriate in different circumstances. Safety and effective treatment must be your primary objectives.

KEY MESSAGE

Your scope of practice extends to treatment techniques that you have been trained to use. Do not undertake treatments for which you are not trained. It is your responsibility to request regular exposure to treatment techniques that you feel need practice.

ABDOMINAL BREATHING

See Active cycle of breathing techniques.

ACTIVE CYCLE OF BREATHING TECHNIQUES (ACBT)

Cycle of deep breathing exercises (thoracic expansion exercises) and huffing (forced expiration technique – FET) interspersed with breathing control, used to aid clearance of secretions. Individual components can be used separately or emphasized within the cycle, depending on the patient's predominant symptoms. May be used in conjunction with other treatments, e.g. manual techniques, positioning.

ACBT – BREATHING CONTROL (BC) (DIAPHRAGMATIC BREATHING, ABDOMINAL BREATHING) (Table 19.1)

Tidal breathing, i.e. not deep breathing. The upper chest and shoulders should be relaxed.

Helpful hints/troubleshooting

● Encourage patients to breathe in through their nose (if appropriate) and to breathe out gently.

Table 19.1 Notes on ACBT – breathing control

	Adult	Child/baby
Indications	● Increased WOB ● Shortness of breath ● Altered breathing pattern ● Panic attacks/anxiety ● Hyperventilation	● Children as adult. May not cooperate ● Babies n/a
Contraindications	● None	● None
Precautions	● Ensure patient is in a comfortable, well-supported position (see Positions of ease) ● Check that the patient is not actively contracting their abdominals – movement of the abdomen should be passive	● As adult

- A hand on the patient's abdomen can check for the desired rise and fall of the abdomen on inspiration and expiration. Be aware that for patients with less effective diaphragmatic activity this movement will be reduced.
- Use your calmest, most relaxing manner (see Relaxation techniques).
- Ensure relaxation of the head, shoulder girdle and thorax.
- Give lots of encouragement, reassurance and praise.
- Do not expect fast results – patients who are experiencing shortness of breath are usually reluctant and/or unable (especially chronic chest patients) to change their breathing pattern quickly.
- Do not insist that the patient abandons bad breathing habits if the patient says they are helping.
- Do not tell patient to 'relax' or 'slow down their breathing' as this may increase anxiety.

ACBT – THORACIC EXPANSION EXERCISES (TEEs) (DEEP BREATHING EXERCISES, LATERAL COSTAL BREATHING) (Table 19.2)

Maximal breath in followed by relaxed expiration. May be used in conjunction with manual techniques (e.g. percussion, vibrations or shaking) or inspiratory hold and/or sniff.

- Inspiratory hold: breath-holding for a few seconds at the end of a deep breath in.
- Sniff: sniffing air in through the nose at the end of a deep breath in with the aim of recruiting collateral ventilation.

Table 19.2 Notes on ACBT – thoracic expansion exercises

	Adult	Child/baby
Indications	● Poor expansion due to collapse ● Sputum retention or atelectasis, pain, fear of pain or immobility	● Children as adult ● Babies n/a
Contraindications	● None	● None
Precautions	● Ensure that the patient has received adequate analgesia, if appropriate, before commencing treatment ● Ensure that the patient is in a suitable position (see Positioning to increase volume)	● As adult

Table 19.3 Notes on ACBT – forced expiration technique

	Adult	Child/baby
Indications	● Sputum retention	● Children as adult ● Babies n/a
Contraindications	● None	● None
Precautions	● Bronchospasm	● As adult

Helpful hints/troubleshooting

● Use your hands to give firm support on the lateral aspects of the patient's ribcage (above the level of rib 8) to monitor the patient's performance and give some sensory input.
● Give lots of encouragement.
● Do not place your hands directly over an incision or painful area of the chest unless the patient is happy for you to do so.
● Do not ask the patient to perform more than three or four deep breaths at a time (may get dizzy).
● Patients who are breathless will not be able to perform consecutive TEEs. Intersperse TEEs with regular breathing control.

ACBT – FORCED EXPIRATION TECHNIQUE (FET) (HUFF) (Table 19.3)

Gentle but forced breath out through an open mouth, following a breath in. The size of breath in will determine the level at which sputum clearance occurs.

19

Helpful hints/troubleshooting

● Spend time making sure the patient understands how to perform the technique effectively.

● Use analogies like 'steam up a mirror' to help your explanation.

● Encourage the patient to huff from a low lung volume, i.e. 'a small breath in' or 'half a breath in' initially, to mobilize peripheral secretions.

● Encourage the patient to huff from larger lung volumes, i.e. 'a deep breath in' to mobilize secretions in more proximal airways.

● The use of different lung volumes may help patients with overwhelming sputum production.

● Huff should be long enough to clear secretions – not simply a clearing of the throat, yet not so long as to lead into paroxysmal coughing.

● Intersperse forced expiration technique with breathing control.

● It can be difficult to teach children this technique. Try using peak flow mouthpiece or blowing games.

ACAPELLA

See Adjuncts.

ADJUNCTS (Table 19.4)

● Acapella

● Cornet (RC-Cornet®)

● Flutter

● PEP mask (positive expiratory pressure mask)

Devices which can be used alone or in conjunction with other techniques in the treatment of retained secretions. Exhalation results in positive expiratory pressure +/– vibration within the airways (no vibration with PEP mask). Only consider using in an on call setting if you are familiar with the techniques and they are regularly used within your Trust.

Table 19.4 Notes on adjuncts

	Adult	Child/baby
Indications	● Sputum retention	● Children as adult ● Babies n/a
Precautions	● None	● Younger children may dislike sealed mask
Contraindications	● None	● None

Helpful hints/troubleshooting

- Not first-line emergency treatment, but do allow patients to use the adjunct if they have already been given one and feel it is helpful.
- In an acute exacerbation some chronic sputum producers, e.g. cystic fibrosis or bronchiectasis, may need some extra help with sputum clearance – this is best discussed with the patient/carers/medical team.
- Allow the patient to hold the device themselves and make sure they maintain an airtight seal.
- Treatment length is approximately 15 minutes and FET is used intermittently.
- It is not possible to breathe in through a Cornet or Flutter.
- With Flutter, make sure that maximal oscillation is achieved by adjusting the angle at which it is held.
- With PEP mask, if a manometer is used the pressure should be between 10 and 20 cmH$_2$O during mid-expiration. A mouthpiece with nose clip may be used instead of a PEP mask.

AUTOGENIC DRAINAGE (Table 19.5)

A technique which mobilizes secretions by using breathing at different lung volumes to produce high airflow in the airways. Needs to be taught to patients by physiotherapists who have had specific training in the technique.

Not a suitable technique to begin teaching in an on call situation, although some patients needing emergency physiotherapy may have been taught it previously. Do not attempt to instruct a patient in this technique unless you have been trained to do so.

Helpful hints/troubleshooting

- Only allow the patient to use this technique in the on call situation if they normally use it independently and they feel it is helpful.

Table 19.5 Notes on autogenic drainage

	Adult	Child/baby
Indications	• Sputum retention • Taught particularly to patients with chronic lung pathology	• Children as adult • Babies n/a
Contraindications	• None	• None
Precautions	• None	• None

19

BAGGING (MANUAL HYPERINFLATION) (Table 19.6)

Deep breaths delivered manually to a mechanically ventilated patient by means of a rebreathing bag.

Slow deep inspiration will offer best physiological benefit (recruit collateral ventilation, improve re-expansion and ABGs). An inspiratory hold at full inspiration will further recruit collateral ventilation (this is not helpful in patients prone to air trapping, e.g. emphysema). A fast expiratory release will mimic FET and may stimulate a cough.

It may be possible to maintain PEEP either held by hand or by means of a PEEP valve – do not try this in an on call siuation unless you have been trained.

Helpful hints/troubleshooting

- Some units may have a policy of using ventilator-delivered inspiratory holds and sighs instead of manual hyperinflation. Check your unit policy before undertaking.
- Use a 2 L bag for adults, a 500 ml open-ended bag for babies, 1 L bag for children.
- Paediatric bags have an open end valve – you will need to practise the technique of effectively and safely bagging this client group.
- Use a manometer when bagging paediatric patients – give approximately 10% above ventilator setting – positive inspiratory pressure/positive end expiratory pressure (PIP/PEEP).
- Do not bag a paediatric patient if you are inexperienced with this age group.
- If you are not confident bagging any patient ask the nurse to assist you by bagging while you undertake physiotherapy. This is a very appropriate use of resources.
- If possible, position the patient with the area of atelectasis or sputum retention uppermost. Side-lying is often the most appropriate position, but not always possible to achieve.
- Watch the patient's chest to assess expansion.
- Coordinate the procedure with the patient's own breathing if they are able to cooperate.
- Stop when audible secretions are heard.
- Do not give more than eight hyperinflations in succession; aim to mimic ACBT with no more than three or four.
- Do not continue if patient shows signs of distress, systolic blood pressure drops below 80 mmHg (55 mmHg in infants, and 75 mmHg in children over 2 years), arrhythmias develop or ICP increases beyond limits set by neurosurgeon or intensivist.

Table 19.6 Notes on bagging

	Adult	Child/baby
Indications	● Intubated patients with atelectasis or sputum retention	● As adults ● Hypoxia
Contraindications	● Undrained pneumothorax ● CVS instability/arrhythmias ● Systolic BP <80 mmHg ● Severe bronchospasm ● Peak airway pressure >40 cmH$_2$O when mechanically ventilated ● High PEEP requirement >15 cmH$_2$O ● Unexplained haemoptysis ● Raised ICP above the set limits	● Undrained pneumothorax ● CVS instability/arrhythmias ● Systolic BP <55 mmHg (infants) or <75 mmHg (children over 2 years) ● Severe bronchospasm ● Severe CVS instability ● Some cardiac conditions ● Raised ICP above the set limits
Precautions	● Use a manometer to monitor peak pressures if available. Do not exceed 40 cmH$_2$O pressure ● PEEP >10 cmH$_2$O – only bag if essential. Use PEEP valve while bagging if patient is PEEP dependent ● Drained pneumothorax ● Recent lung surgery (within last 14 days) ● Arrhythmias or unstable BP ● On 100% O$_2$ (FiO$_2$ = 1) – disconnection from the ventilator may cause sudden desaturation ● Watch the monitor for changes in heart rate or blood pressure ● Reduced respiratory drive – an air/oxygen mix may be preferable ● Raised ICP within the set limits	● High-frequency oscillation – leave on ventilator as much as possible ● Labile BP ● Watch volume and pressure as pneumothorax easily happens ● Raised ICP within the set limits

BREATHING CONTROL

See Active cycle of breathing techniques.

CORNET (RC-CORNET®)

See Adjuncts.

COUGH (Table 19.7)

Reflex or voluntary mechanism for clearing airways of secretions or foreign body. An effective breath in and closure of the glottis is required to generate enough expiratory velocity to create an effective cough; some patients may not be able to do this. Manual support from therapist's hands or a pillow over incision or painful area such as fractured ribs can increase effectiveness.

Helpful hints/troubleshooting

- Ensure adequate pain relief has been given before commencing treatment.
- Allow the patient to sip a hot or cold drink intermittently during treatment if mouth is dry. For patients who are NBM let patient use mouthwash or suck an ice cube.
- Ensure the patient is in a well-supported position and leaning forward if possible, or with their knees drawn up towards their chest.
- Do not insist on repeated coughing if the patient is not productive.

Table 19.7 Notes on cough

	Adult	Child/baby
Indications	● Prevention and treatment of sputum retention	● Children as adult ● Babies n/a
Contraindications	● None	● As adult
Precautions	● Pain – ensure adequate analgesia ● Severe bronchospasm – avoid paroxysmal coughing ● Discourage unnecessary coughing in patients with significant frank haemoptysis, bleeding oesophageal varices, raised ICP either measured or suspected or recent cerebral bleed, major eye surgery	● Pertussis (whooping cough) – paroxysmal coughing can cause severe desaturation and bradycardia

Table 19.8 Notes on assisted cough

	Adult	Child/baby
Indications	● Prevention and treatment of sputum retention	● Children as adult ● Useful in children with degenerative neuromuscular disorders, e.g. Duchenne muscular dystrophy ● Babies n/a
Contraindications	● Pressure on abdomen should be avoided as below; direct pressure over rib fractures of chest wall injuries/incisions should be avoided	● As adult
Precautions	● Immediately following surgery, especially post upper abdominal surgery, eye surgery, cardiothoracic surgery ● Paralytic ileus ● Rib fractures ● Raised intracranial pressure ● Undrained pneumothorax ● Osteoporosis ● Pain ● Unstable spine – an appropriate hold must be used to counter any movement	● As adult

Assisted cough (Table 19.8)

Manual upwards compression of diaphragm given by therapist to replace the work of the abdominals in order to facilitate a cough in patients with spinal cord injury or neuromuscular disease (Fig. 19.1).

Helpful hints/troubleshooting

● If one person is assisting – place one hand on near side of chest and the other on the opposite side with the forearm resting on the lower ribs (Fig. 19.1a).
● As the patient coughs the physiotherapist pushes in and up with the forearm and stabilizes the thorax with the hands.
● Or (Fig. 19.1b) both hands are placed on the lower thorax, with the elbows extended, and the physiotherapist pushes in and up with both arms.
● In large patients or with very tenacious sputum two people (Fig. 19.1d) may be needed to assist effectively.

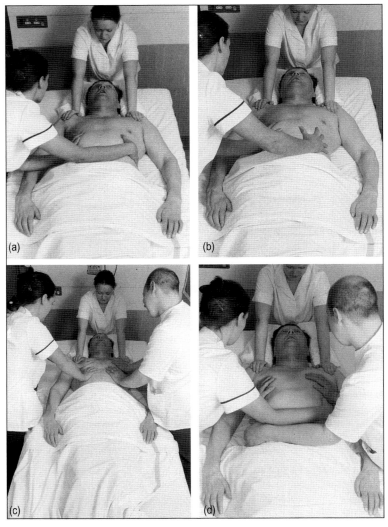

Figure 19.1 Assisted coughing. Reproduced from Pryor and Prasad (2002), with kind permission.

● Care is needed to synchronize the assisted cough with the patient's attempt to cough.
● Pressure should be released as soon as the cough is over.
● Patients with long-term cough assistance needs may have developed an effective interpretation of the above.

COUGH ASSIST DEVICE (MANUAL INSUFFLATION/EXSUFFLATION)
(Table 19.9)

Device which assists cough effort by means of a positive pressure breath followed by a rapid switch to negative pressure. Most effective in patients who have an ineffective cough due to neuromuscular weakness. However, increasing use with other groups of patients.

Helpful hints/troubleshooting

● Fear, pain and poor technique will lead to poor synchrony with the machine and an ineffective treatment.
● A tight seal is essential – use either a face mask or a mouthpiece with nose clip; coughing is easier with a face mask if tolerated.
● Use as established with the patient – either the operator will synchronize the breath in and breath out to negative pressure with the patient, or the automatic mode may be used.
● Start with a low inspiratory pressure, e.g. 10 cmH$_2$O, and gradually raise the pressure to achieve a deep breath with the patient (if on NIV start at the level set on the ventilator); initially keep inspiratory and expiratory pressure equal. Then increase expiratory pressure if the patient needs more 'suck'. Refer to your unit policy.
● The patient is instructed to cough when the breath out starts.
● The technique can be combined with an assisted cough.
● The patient may need a few inspiratory breaths post coughing to recover.

Table 19.9 Notes on cough assist device

	Adult	**Child/baby**
Indications	● Prevention and treatment of sputum retention	● Children as adult ● Babies n/a
Contraindications	● Undrained pneumothorax	● As adult
Precautions	● Oxygen dependency; entrain oxygen into the breathing circuit ● Do not instigate use in the on call setting if you are not fully trained and confident ● Bronchospasm	● As adult

19

COUGH STIMULATION/TRACHEAL RUB

This is a highly contentious issue – only use the technique if you are trained in its use and it is accepted practice within your unit.

CONTINUOUS POSITIVE AIRWAY PRESSURE (CPAP) (Table 19.10)

Continuous positive pressure delivered throughout inspiration and expiration administered to a spontaneously breathing patient. Requires a high oxygen flow rate, delivered via an airtight mask, mouthpiece (with nose clip), tracheostomy or ET tube (Fig. 19.2). Can be given periodically or continuously.

Table 19.10 Notes on CPAP

	Adult	Child/baby
Indications	● Increased WOB or hypoxaemia caused by atelectasis, reduced FRC, flail chest, poor gas exchange across the basement membrane due to inflammation, pulmonary oedema, chronic damage	● As adults
Contraindications	● Undrained pneumothorax ● Frank haemoptysis ● Vomiting ● Facial fractures, nasal approach for neurosurgery ● CVS instability ● Raised ICP ● Recent upper GI surgery ● Active TB ● Lung abscess	● As adults
Precautions	● Increasing $PaCO_2$ ● Emphysema – check CXR for large bullae ● Patient compliance ● Skin around mask can break down easily ● Patients with airways obstructed by a tumour – may cause air trapping ● Deranged platelets	● As adults. Children tend to dislike the sealed mask ● Watch the amount of CPAP given – too much can cause increased WOB ● Start at 4 cmH_2O and assess patient closely

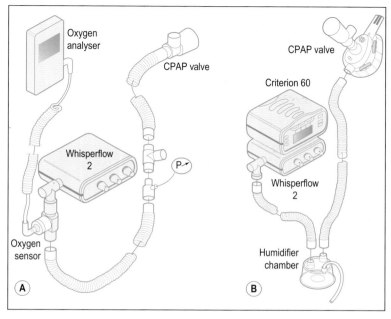

Figure 19.2 Diagram to show an example of a CPAP circuit. Reproduced with the kind permission of Profile Systems Ltd.

Helpful hints/troubleshooting

● Oxygen and pressure levels should be set in liaison with medical staff. Do not try to set up this equipment unless you have been shown how to do so. Ask for assistance from ICU.

● Patients on CPAP generally require higher dependency care – check hospital policy with the ward sister.

● Other types of treatment such as breathing exercises can still be used with patients who are breathing with the assistance of CPAP. Monitor the patient's oxygen saturation if you need to remove the patient's mask for any reason, e.g. in order for them to cough.

● The beneficial effects of the CPAP are lost within minutes of removal – thus it may be in the patient's best interests to stay on CPAP. However, it may be appropriate, once stabilized, to enable the patient to have short periods of time without the CPAP for personal hygiene, skin care and a drink.

● Humidification is recommended.

● Be aware that CPAP will not correct a climbing $PaCO_2$ in adults, but can sometimes be effective in infants under 1 year old.

DEEP BREATHING EXERCISES

See Active cycle of breathing techniques.

DIAPHRAGMATIC BREATHING

See Active cycle of breathing techniques.

FLUTTER

See Adjuncts.

FORCED EXPIRATION TECHNIQUE (FET)

See Active cycle of breathing techniques.

GRAVITY-ASSISTED POSITIONING/DRAINAGE

See Positioning.

HUFF

See Active cycle of breathing techniques – FET.

HUMIDIFICATION (Table 19.11)

Inhaled water vapour or aerosol administered by mask.

Table 19.11 Notes on humidification

	Adult	Child/baby
Indications	● Sputum retention, particularly thick sticky secretions, difficulty expectorating, dry mouth ● Patients needing continuous oxygen (oxygen is a dry gas) ● Patients breathing via a tracheostomy/ET tube (the natural warming mechanism of the nasal passages is bypassed)	● As adult
Contraindications	● None	● None
Precautions	● Patients prone to bronchospasm may react to nebulized water. Use saline if required – this will reduce the lifespan of the humidification unit as the saline will crystallize ● Airway/facial burns if heated humidification is unmonitored (all new equipment should have temperature gauges and alarms)	● Can exacerbate fluid overload in cardiac conditions ● Given via head box in infants and mask in children

Helpful hints/troubleshooting

● Many different types of equipment available. Make sure you are familiar with the type your unit uses.

● Using the bubble-through method to humidify via nasal cannulae will return gas to atmospheric humidification but will not increase it; the water tends to condense in the narrow tubing. Wide diameter tubing and mask are essential for effective delivery.

● Give humidification time to have an effect. Ideally, if indicated, ask for it to be commenced before you arrive on the scene. If you commence humidification as part of your treatment allow approximately 10–15 minutes before recommencing sputum clearance techniques.

● Cold air blowing onto heated humidification tubing (e.g. fans, open windows) will cause water to collect in the tubing – this should be emptied regularly and ideally avoided, if necessary by turning the temperature down.

● Due to the potential for infection, humidification units should not be left switched off and then reused.

● Also consider regular prescribed saline nebulizers (usually 5 ml of 0.9% saline) and appropriate systemic hydration.

INCENTIVE SPIROMETER (Table 19.12)

Device which gives visual feedback on performance of slow deep breath in.

Helpful hints/troubleshooting

● Give clear instructions. Patients need to be able to remember how to use the device so that they can use it when you are not there.

● Encourage the patient to adopt a position which will facilitate deep breathing (see Positioning to increase volume).

● Be aware that patients can quickly learn to cheat – ensure that what you are seeing is indeed the product of a slow deep breath in.

Table 19.12 Notes on incentive spirometer

	Adult	Child/baby
Indications	● Volume loss. May be useful for patients who have difficulty with understanding the concept of TEEs	● Children as adult. Limited to use by older children ● Babies n/a
Contraindications	● None	● None
Precautions	● None	● None

19

- Unhelpful for patients who are breathless.
- Cannot be used with patients who require a high concentration of continuous oxygen by mask.

INTERMITTENT POSITIVE PRESSURE BREATHING (IPPB) (Table 19.13)

Device (e.g. 'Bird', Bennett PR2) which delivers positive pressure on inspiration only, to increase tidal volume and rest respiratory muscles; delivery is by mouthpiece or face mask (Fig. 19.3).

Helpful hints/troubleshooting

- Position the patient so that the affected lung is uppermost, if applicable.
- Adult settings for IPPB where numbered dials are present:
  - Sensitivity – keep low at approx 7, unless the machine appears to be triggering too easily.
  - Flow rate – start at 10 unless patient is very breathless. If very SOB start higher (over 20) and be prepared quickly to adjust it until the breath in is fast enough for the patient.

Table 19.13 Notes on IPPB

	Adult	Child/baby
Indications	• Increased WOB, sputum retention, poor tidal volume particularly in weak or tired patients	• As adult • Children older than 6 years of age seem to be able to comply
Contraindications	• Undrained pneumothorax • Frank haemoptysis • Vomiting blood (haematemesis) • Facial fractures, nasal approach for neurosurgery • CVS instability • Raised ICP • Recent lung/upper GI surgery • Active TB • Lung abscess	• As adult
Precautions	• Emphysema – check CXR for bullae • Patients with airways obstructed by a tumour – may cause air trapping • Deranged platelets	• As adult

19

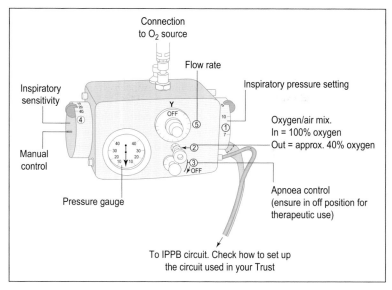

Figure 19.3 Diagram to show an example of IPPB dials.

- ● Pressure – start at 10 and aim to increase as able within the limits of the patient during the treatment.
- ● In paediatric patients, DO NOT use if the patient is uncompliant or under 5 years old.
- ● Suggested starting pressures for paediatric patients: 10 cmH$_2$O then increase to 20–25 cmH$_2$O maximum.
- ● Pay attention to ensuring that after triggering the machine the rest of the inspiratory phase is passive – the patient must allow the machine to do the work of inspiration.
- ● Ensure that the patient is reaching the set pressure. If the pressure dial swings above the set pressure level, it is likely that the patient is blowing out into the machine – the machine will cut out early and the set pressure will not actually be achieved.
- ● Use 0.9% saline in the machine's nebulizer.
- ● An effective seal is essential, either by means of a tight seal with the face mask (you will need to make sure that the head is supported so that you can hold the mask securely in place), or use a mouthpiece and pinch the nose. A nose clip may be useful for some patients.

- Use for short periods of time, not continuously, e.g. 10 minutes every hour. Remember not to give the patient more than about four to eight big breaths in a row. If the nursing staff are to assist the patient it is essential that they are familiar with the equipment, the risk of pneumothorax, and are aware not to change the settings.
- Do not allow the patient to use the machine unsupervised unless you are confident they can use it effectively.
- If everything is going wrong and you lose confidence with the Bird as you start your treatment, take the machine away and, with a clean circuit, use the machine on yourself to sort out the cause of any problem, then return to the patient and start again.

LATERAL COSTAL BREATHING
See Active cycle of breathing techniques.

MANUAL HYPERINFLATION
See Bagging.

MOBILIZATION (Table 19.14)
Assisted walking or other functional activity such as moving from bed to chair. Most patients requiring on call physiotherapy will not be well enough to mobilize, but it may be necessary to help them move in order to get the patient into a more appropriate position for treatment.

Helpful hints/troubleshooting
- Ensure you get sufficient help before attempting to help a patient get out of bed.
- Work with the patient enabling them to assist in the manoeuvre as much as possible.
- The child in pain will be reluctant to mobilize. Ensure adequate analgesia and utilize all your powers of persuasion and bribery!

NEUROPHYSIOLOGICAL FACILITATION OF RESPIRATION
The selective use of external proprioceptive and tactile stimuli to produce a reflex respiratory response, with the aim of improving an aspect of ventilatory activity. These techniques are appropriate for on call treatments only if you are familiar with their effective use.

19

Table 19.14 Notes on mobilization

	Adult	Child/baby
Indications	● Sputum retention ● Volume loss ● Limited to previously mobile patients	● Children as adult ● A toddler may need assistance to mobilize ● Babies – ensure that the baby is able to roll and move around the cot – THIS IS STILL MOBILIZING THE PATIENT!
Contraindications	● CVS instability ● Low BP, serious arrhythmia	● As adult
Precautions	● Drips, drains and catheters ● Ensure pain controlled ● Follow local protocols for patients with epidural analgesia or post orthopaedic, plastic and vascular surgery	● As adult

NON-INVASIVE VENTILATION (NIV) (Table 19.15)

Device which provides ventilatory support by delivering a pre-set volume or pressure by mask either automatically or in response to patient's inspiratory effort. Some machines are able to add positive end expiratory pressure. Do not set up NIV unless you are familiar with the equipment and are confident as to how safely to establish the patient on NIV and appropriately respond to blood gas results.

Helpful hints/troubleshooting

● The decision to use NIV and the settings chosen must always be made with the medical and nursing team looking after the patient.
● Introduce the treatment to the patient slowly.
● Patient needs to keep mouth closed if using nasal mask.
● Some patients are less suited to NIV; however, each situation should be individually assessed.
● NIV should generally be used in ICU/HDU environments – make sure you are aware of your local policy.

19

Table 19.15 Notes on NIV

	Adult	Child/baby
Indications	● Increased WOB causing ventilatory failure, i.e. increased CO_2, fatigue, neuromuscular disorders	● As adult ● Not often used in infants – nasal CPAP more commonly used
Contraindications	● Undrained pneumothorax ● Frank haemoptysis ● Vomiting blood (haematemesis) ● Facial fractures ● CVS instability ● Raised ICP ● Recent upper GI surgery ● Active TB ● Lung abscess	● As adults
Precautions	● Emphysema – check CXR for bullae ● Patient compliance ● Skin around mask can break down easily ● Patients with airways obstructed by a tumour – may cause air trapping	● As adults ● Children may dislike the tight sealed mask

The steps in initiating NIV therapy

(Reproduced from Pryor and Prasad (2002), with kind permission)

● Introduce the patient slowly to the equipment and all its parts.
● Ensure the mask fits comfortably and that the patient can experience the mask on their face without the ventilator connected.
● Allow the patient the opportunity to feel the operation of the machine through the mask on their hand or cheek before applying it over their nose or mouth.
● Allow the patient the opportunity to practise breathing with the ventilator, either holding the mask in place or allowing them to hold it in place before applying the straps.
● Adjust settings initially for comfort and establish whether the patient can relax comfortably in a sleeping posture.
● Provide opportunities for the patient to feed back any discomfort or uncertainty with regard to the use of the equipment.
● Assess and adjust the performance of the ventilator during an afternoon nap to optimize gas exchange and patient comfort.
● Progress to an overnight study, continuing to monitor and optimize gas exchange and sleep quality.

Characteristics of patients with acute respiratory failure unlikely to do well on NIV

(Reproduced from Pryor and Prasad (2002), with kind permission)

- Agitation, encephalopathic, uncooperative
- Severe illness, including extreme acidosis (pH <7.2)
- Presence of excessive secretions or pneumonia
- Multiple organ failure
- Haemodynamic instability
- Inability to maintain a lip seal
- Inability to protect the airway
- Overt respiratory failure requiring immediate intubation.

OVERPRESSURE

Applied at the end of the breath out and is quickly released to stimulate inspiration. Care is needed in patients with chest trauma/post surgery and fragile ribs, e.g. osteoporosis.

OXYGEN THERAPY (Table 19.16)

Delivery of higher concentration of oxygen than is present in room air, i.e. 24–100% by mask. Should be prescribed in writing by a doctor in adults but given as necessary without prescription in paediatrics unless there is an underlying duct-dependent cardiac lesion. Any change (beyond appropriate pre-oxygenation for suction) must be discussed with the medical team.

Give the minimum dose necessary to have the effect you want, since oxygen is potentially toxic if given without need in high concentrations over a prolonged period.

Table 19.16 Notes on oxygen therapy

	Adult	Child/baby
Indications	● Hypoxaemia ● Before and after suction	● As adult
Contraindications	● None	● Duct-dependent cardiac lesions – follow local protocols
Precautions	● Hypercapnic COPD patients who may be dependent on hypoxaemia for respiratory drive – use ABGs to assess (see Chapter 3)	● Remember humidification via head box or mask if over 2 L/min

19

Table 19.17 Notes on percussion

	Adult	Child/baby
Indications	● Sputum retention	● As adult
Contraindications	● Directly over rib fracture ● Directly over a surgical incision or graft ● Frank haemoptysis ● Severe osteoporosis	● Hypoxia – percussion can exacerbate hypoxia, especially in infants
Precautions	● Profound hypoxaemia ● Bronchospasm, pain ● Osteoporosis, bony metastases ● Near chest drains	● As adult ● **Baby – make sure head is supported**

Helpful hints/troubleshooting
● Ensure adequate humidification is provided with continuous use of high concentrations.
● Avoid prolonged patient exposure to unnecessarily high concentrations.

PEP MASK (POSITIVE EXPIRATORY PRESSURE MASK)
See Adjuncts.

PERCUSSION (Table 19.17)
Rhythmic clapping on the patient's chest with cupped hands or soft-rimmed face mask.

Helpful hints/troubleshooting
● For adults and older children perform in conjunction with thoracic expansion exercises.
● To minimize hypoxaemia percussion during TEEs (i.e. approximately 30 seconds) is recommended.
● Cushion the patient with a folded towel, and be careful not to be heavy handed – patient comfort is important.

POSITIONING: POSITIONS OF EASE
Well-supported patient positions used with spontaneously breathing patients which encourage relaxation of the upper chest and shoulders (Fig. 19.4 and Table 19.18).

POSITIONING: POSTURAL DRAINAGE (GRAVITY-ASSISTED DRAINAGE)
Positions which allow gravity to help drain retained secretions (Figs 19.5 and 19.6, and Tables 19.19 and 19.20).

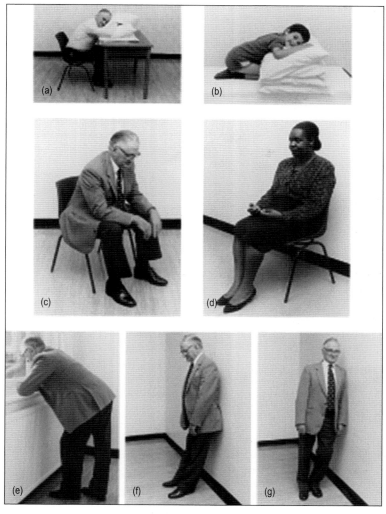

Figure 19.4 Positions of ease. (a) Forward-lean sitting. (b) Forward kneeling. (c, d) Relaxed sitting. (e) Forward-lean standing. (f, g) Relaxed standing. Reproduced from Pryor and Prasad (2002), with kind permission.

Table 19.18 Notes on positions of ease

	Adult	Child/baby
Indications	● Increased WOB ● SOB at rest and on exercise ● Anxiety/panic attacks ● Hyperventilation	● Children as adult ● Babies (see Fig. 19.5a)
Contraindications	● None	● None
Precautions	● None	● None

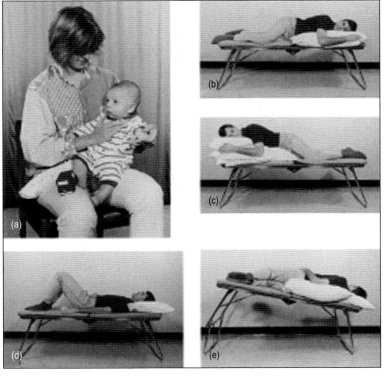

Figure 19.5 Postural drainage. (a) Apical segments, upper lobes. (b) Posterior segment, right upper lobe. (c) Posterior segment, left upper lobe. (d) Anterior segments, upper lobes. (e) Lingula. Reproduced from Pryor and Prasad (2002), with kind permission.

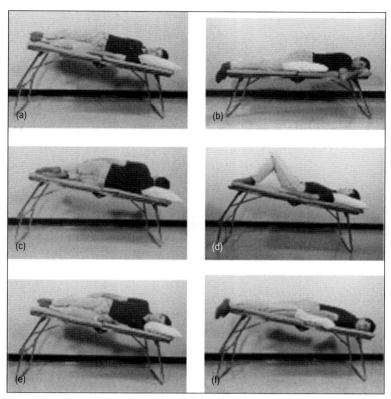

Figure 19.6 Postural drainage. (a) Right middle lobe. (b) Apical segments, lower lobes. (c) Right medial basal and left lateral basal segments, lower lobes. (d) Anterior basal segments. (e) Lateral basal segment, right lower lobe. (f) Posterior basal segments, lower lobes. Reproduced from Pryor and Prasad (2002), with kind permission.

Table 19.19 Notes on postural drainage

	Adult	Child/baby
Indications	● Sputum retention, particularly if localized to one lung segment or lobe	● As adult

Table 19.19 *Continued*

	Adult	Child/baby
Contraindications to head-down position	● Hypertension ● Severe dyspnoea ● Recent surgery ● Severe haemoptysis ● Nose bleeds ● Advanced pregnancy ● Hiatus hernia ● Cardiac failure ● Cerebral oedema ● Aortic aneurysm ● Head or neck trauma/surgery ● Mechanical ventilation	● As adult
Precautions	● Diaphragmatic paralysis/weakness	● Head-down position can cause reflux, vomiting and aspiration, and splints the diaphragm reducing respiratory effectiveness

Table 19.20 Gravity-assisted drainage positions (Prasad and Pryor 2002)

	Lobe	Position
Upper lobe	● Apical bronchus ● Posterior bronchus ● Right ● Left ● Anterior bronchus	● Sitting upright ● Lying on the left side horizontally turned 45° on to the face, resting against a pillow, with another supporting the head ● Lying on the right side turned 45° on to the face, with three pillows arranged to lift the shoulders 30 cm from the horizontal ● Lying supine with the knees flexed
Lingula	● Superior brochus ● Inferior bronchus	● Lying supine with the body a quarter turned to the right maintained by a pillow under the left side from shoulder to hip. The chest is tilted downwards to an angle of 15°
Middle lobe	● Lateral bronchus ● Medial bronchus	● Lying supine with the body a quarter turned to the left maintained by a pillow under the right side from shoulder to hip. The chest is tilted downwards to an angle of 15°

Table 19.20 *Continued*

	Lobe	Position
Lower lobe	● Apical bronchus ● Medial basal (cardiac) bronchus ● Anterior basal bronchus ● Lateral basal bronchus ● Posterior basal bronchus	● Lying prone with a pillow under the abdomen ● Lying on the right side with the chest tilted downwards to an angle of 20° ● Lying supine with the knees flexed and the chest tilted downwards to an angle of 20° ● Lying on the opposite side with the chest tilted downwards to an angle of 20° ● Lying prone with a pillow under the hips and the chest tilted downwards to an angle of 20°

Helpful hints/troubleshooting

● Do not use head-down tilt immediately after meals/feed.
● Position needs to be maintained for at least 10 minutes to achieve a beneficial effect.
● Can be modified to side-lying (affected lung uppermost) with or without head-down tip for more generalized secretions or those with contraindications to head-down position.
● Drain worst affected area first.
● Most hospital beds have a catch at the bottom of the bed or an electric switch which will tip the bed feet up.
● Especially in children positioning for drainage may result in a V/Q mismatch. Discuss this with the medical team. It may be necessary either to adapt the position or temporarily to increase the oxygen.

POSITIONING TO INCREASE VOLUME (Table 19.21)

Positioning of spontaneously breathing patients to facilitate maximal inspiration. Use the most upright position that the patient can tolerate, e.g. standing, high sitting; otherwise side-lying is an acceptable alternative.

Helpful hints/troubleshooting

● Get as much help as you need to move the patient safely.

POSITIONING TO MATCH VENTILATION/PERFUSION RATIO (Table 19.22)

Positioning which attempts maximally to perfuse and ventilate the same area of healthy lung tissue. Best applied to patients with unilateral pathology.

19

Table 19.21 Notes on positioning to increase volume

	Adult	Child/baby
Indications	● Volume loss, i.e. poor expansion due to pain, fear of pain, immobility	● As adult
Contraindications	● CVS instability ● Unstable spinal fracture ● Unstable head injury	● As adult
Precautions	● Proceed slowly if standing the patient for the first time after a period of bed rest	● As adult

Table 19.22 Notes on positioning to match ventilation/perfusion ratio

	Adult	Child/baby
Indications	● Hypoxaemia	● As adult
Contraindications	● As above (Table 19.21)	● As adult
Precautions	● As above	● As adult
Ventilated	● Lung with pathology down	● Lung with pathology up (baby and small child)
Non-ventilated	● Lung with pathology up	● Lung with pathology down (baby and small child)

Helpful hints/troubleshooting
● Get as much help as you need to move the patient safely.
● Ensure that you are happy with principles of ventilation and perfusion before deciding how to position the patient – dependent regions of lung are preferentially ventilated and perfused in spontaneously breathing adults.
● Babies, small children and mechanically ventilated adults ventilate non-dependent lung regions while perfusing dependent regions and it is therefore difficult to match ventilation and perfusion.

POSITIONING: PRONE

Profoundly hypoxic patients may be nursed prone as this aids the recruitment of lung tissue. Chest physiotherapy is still possible in this position if appropriate. Most patients requiring this intervention do not have sputum retention as a problem; they require high levels of PEEP and oxygen and may thus not benefit from physiotherapy. Be aware of the need to protect neural and soft tissues when positioning. Figure 19.7C illustrates the recommended upper limb position, but

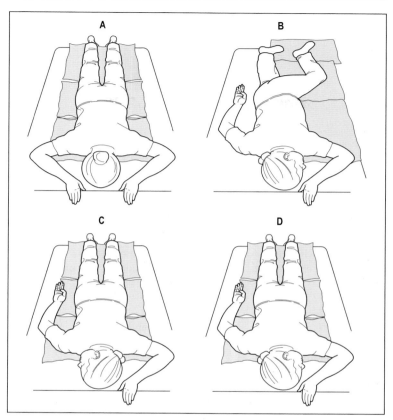

Figure 19.7A–D Diagram to show recommended prone position (B) and suggested modifications (A and C) according to patient's shape, pressure area care and need to protect neuromusculoskeletal structures. Adapted from Ball et al (2001), with kind permission.

this may need to be modified (as shown in Fig. 19.7A, B or D) to suit the needs of individual patients; check with local Trust or unit policy.

This position is used commonly in paediatrics due to its beneficial effect on gas exchange. If you utilize this position, make sure that the patient is carefully monitored (i.e. HR, BP, SpO_2, RR) owing to the link with sudden infant death syndrome.

POSITIVE EXPIRATORY PRESSURE MASK
See Adjuncts.

19

Table 19.23 Notes on relaxation techniques

	Adult	Child/baby
Indications	● Increased WOB ● SOB at rest and on exercise ● Altered breathing pattern ● Panic attacks, anxiety ● Hyperventilation	● Children as adult ● Babies n/a
Contraindications	● None	● None
Precautions	● None	● None

POSTURAL DRAINAGE
See Positioning.

RELAXATION TECHNIQUES (Table 19.23)
Techniques which help patients reduce unhelpful muscle tension. May include appropriate use of voice, calm manner, advice on positioning, advice on breathing and specific relaxation techniques such as 'Laura Mitchell', or 'contract/relax'.

Helpful hints/troubleshooting
● Never underestimate the power of relaxation: simple positioning, use of voice and reassurance can have a profound impact upon anxiety-related increased WOB and bronchospasm.
● Ensure that you are relaxed yourself if you intend to try to reduce tension in your patient.
● Position the patient appropriately – forward-lean sitting or high side-lying are useful.
● Incorporate appropriate aspects of relaxation into managing the breathing problem.
● Be aware that a noisy bustling ward will reduce the efficacy of your treatment!

RELAXED TIDAL BREATHING
See Active cycle of breathing techniques.

RIB SPRINGING
Used in the paralysed patient. Compression of the chest wall is continued throughout expiration with the application of overpressure at the end of expiration. A quick release encourages inspiration.

Care is required at the level of compression offered as the patient is unable to report pain. Do not use unless familiar with the technique. Contraindicated for babies and all patients with fragile ribs/vertebrae (e.g. osteoporosis).

SALINE NEBULIZER
See Humidification.

SHAKING (Table 19.24)
Coarse oscillations produced by the therapist's hands compressing and releasing the chest wall. Performed during thoracic expansion exercises, on exhalation only.

Helpful hints/troubleshooting
● Perform on the expiration phase only following a deep breath in.
● Obtain feedback from the patient concerning comfort – this technique should not be uncomfortable.

SPUTUM INDUCTION (INDUCED SPUTUM)
Not generally an indication for emergency physiotherapy. Check if the call out is still appropriate for physiotherapy treatment.

SUCTION
Endotracheal suction (Table 19.25)
Removal of secretions from the upper airways using a suction catheter, in patients who are intubated or have a tracheostomy.

Table 19.24 Notes on shaking

	Adult	Child/baby
Indications	● Sputum retention	● Sputum retention
Contraindications	● Directly over rib fracture or surgical incision	● Premature infants – causes brain injury – DO NOT USE
Precautions	● Long-term oral steroids/ osteoporosis, bony metastases ● Near chest drains ● Severe bronchospasm	● Rib fractures ● **Baby – make sure head is supported**

19

Table 19.25 Notes on endotracheal suction

	Adult	Child/baby

Indications	● Sputum retention in intubated patients
	● Sputum retention may be indicated by high peak airway pressures with volume-controlled ventilation or decreased tidal volume with pressure-controlled ventilation, auscultation, hypoxaemia or reduced SpO_2
	● Visible/audible secretions not effectively removed with a cough and causing respiratory distress
	● Poor cough caused by neurological pathology, pain inhibition, or inhibition by drugs
	● Aspiration
	● Reduced tidal volumes in ventilated patients
	● Increased peak pressures in ventilated patients
		● Sputum retention indicated by increased work of breathing in association with other signs:
		  ● Decreased SpO_2/hypoxia
		  ● Deteriorating blood gases in association with other indications
		  ● Increased HR
		● Auscultation in association with other indications

Contraindications	● None if indicated	● As adult
Precautions	● Low SpO_2 ● Dependency on high O_2 ● High ventilatory requirements (closed circuit catheters will reduce need to disconnect patient from ventilator) ● Severe CVS instability ● Anticoagulated patients or those with clotting disorders ● Severe bronchospasm ● Recent lung oesophageal surgery	● As adult

Helpful hints/troubleshooting

● Preoxygenate before and after suction either by bagging or by increasing the baseline FiO_2 on the ventilator by:
  a. 10% for children/babies
  b. 20% or up to 100% depending upon unit policy for adults.
● Use each catheter only once unless closed system suction is used.
● Discontinue if arrhythmias develop, or HR/BP drops.
● Explain the procedure to the patient with lots of reassurance.

- Guide to suction catheter size:
  a. Paeds – internal diameter of ET or tracheostomy tube in millimetres multiplied by 2, e.g. tube size 3.5 mm × 2 = size 7 (French gauge) suction catheter
  b. Adults internal diameter of ET or tracheostomy tube in millimetres, minus 2 then multiply by 2, e.g. tube size 8 mm − 2 = 6 × 2 = size 12 (French gauge) suction catheter.

Pharyngeal suction (Table 19.26)

Removal of secretions from the upper airways by means of a suction catheter introduced via the nose or mouth. Generally only indicated for patients who are unconscious/semiconscious or neurologically impaired. (See section on consent, Chapter 2, pp 14–16.)

Helpful hints/troubleshooting

- Use an airway for oral suction or frequent nasal suctioning.
- Preoxygenate the patient.
- Position the patient in side-lying in case they vomit.

Table 19.26 Notes on pharyngeal suction

	Adult	Child/baby
Indications	• Retained secretions/ aspiration in the upper airways of patients who are unable to cough or have reduced cough caused by fatigue, neurological pathology, pain inhibition, or inhibition by drugs	• Visible/audible secretions not effectively removed with a cough and causing respiratory distress • Poor cough caused by neurological pathology, pain inhibition, or inhibition by drugs • Aspiration
Contraindications	• Stridor • Skull fractures • Craniofacial surgery/injury	• Haemangioma • As adult
Precautions	• High malignancy, high oesophageal varices • Anticoagulated patients or those with clotting disorders • Severe CVS instability • Severe bronchospasm • Recent pneumonectomy or oesophagectomy – liaise with surgeons	• As adult

19

- Use a 'clean' technique.
- Do not use on any patient who would require physical restraining in order to carry out the procedure.
- Do not suction patients to remove pulmonary oedema as it will be replaced and surfactant will be removed.
- Remember to give the patient lots of reassurance.
- Some units will insert a mini-tracheostomy (a thin blue tube) into the trachea if repeated suction is needed. This procedure is associated with as much risk as formal tracheostomy insertion and thus the decision is not taken lightly. Mini-tracheostomy is not used in the majority of paediatric units.
- Try to avoid using oropharyngeal suction in babies as this increases the risk of vomiting and aspiration.

THORACIC EXPANSION EXERCISES
See Active cycle of breathing techniques.

VIBRATIONS (Table 19.27)
Fine oscillations applied to the chest wall by the therapist's hands or fingertips (in babies). Performed during thoracic expansion exercises, on exhalation only.

Helpful hints/troubleshooting
- Use firm contact and direct the force inwards towards the centre of the patient's chest.
- Perform on the expiration phase only following a deep breath in.

Table 19.27 Notes on vibrations

	Adult	Child/baby
Indications	● Sputum retention	● Sputum retention
Contraindications	● Directly over rib fracture or surgical incision ● Severe bronchospasm	● Premature infants – causes brain injury if head is unsupported
Precautions	● Long-term oral steroids/osteoporosis ● Near chest drains	● Rib fractures ● Make sure head is supported

19

References

Ball C, Adams J, Boyce S et al (2001) Clinical guidelines for the use of the prone position in acute respiratory distress syndrome. Intensive Crit Care Nurs 17(2):94–104.

Pryor JA, Prasad SA (eds) (2002) Physiotherapy for respiratory and cardiac problems,
3rd edn. London: Churchill Livingstone.

Further reading

Hough A (2001) Physiotherapy in respiratory care, 3rd edn. Cheltenham: Stanley
Thornes.

CHAPTER 20

Case studies

This chapter contains a number of case studies written by the authors. Work through the ones specific to your learning needs. Do not worry if the information given or presentation differs – this is all part of the learning process.

CASE STUDY 1: ADULT INTENSIVE CARE
Rachel Devlin and Zoe Van Willigan

History
34-year-old man admitted to ICU following respiratory arrest; admitted 4 days ago for nasogastric feeding.

Past medical history
15-year history of anorexia; previous admissions for nutritional management. Depression

Drug history
Citalopram

Observation/examination
The patient is supine in bed. The nursing staff report the patient only arrived on the unit an hour ago and they have not suctioned him yet. The patient is cachexic; his weight has been estimated at 35 kg.

A: Intubated and ventilated via endotracheal tube

B: PS 25, PEEP 10, RR 30, TV 300 ml, PAP 36
FiO$_2$ 0.6, SpO$_2$ 92%
ABGs: pH 7.36, pCO$_2$ 4.92, pO$_2$ 7.39, HCO$_3$ 22.0, BE −1.0
Ausc.: Decreased air entry throughout right lung
Expansion: left > right
Palpation: Nil

C: HR 100, BP 100/70, Temp. 38°C

Renal: UO 40 ml, Fluid balance +900 ml

D: AVP̲U

Propofol, fentanyl

E: Arterial line, peripheral access, urinary catheter.

You have been asked to see this patient urgently as he was found to have a right-sided 'white out' on the post-intubation CXR.

Questions

1. What is the patient's main problem?
2. What will be your treatment plan?
3. What considerations might you need to take into account prior to treatment?
4. How will you know if your treatment is effective?

Answers

1. Aspiration to the right lung. The patient's NG tube has migrated from his stomach allowing the aspiration of NG feed.
2. Treatment plan:
a. Reposition the patient in left side-lying to aid drainage of secretions.
b. Suction to clear secretions.
c. Manual hyperinflation to reinflate right lung.
3. Considerations:
- **PEEP**: PEEP of >10 cmH$_2$O
- **High PAP**: This patient is requiring high levels of PS and PEEP to maintain adequate gaseous exchange.
- **Low BMI**: Normally a patient will be ventilated to achieve a tidal volume of 6–8 ml per kg. Care needs to be taken with positioning to avoid pressure area problems.
- **Low BP**: This BP may be acceptable for this patient because of his low BMI.
4. Ask for a repeat CXR and ABGs following treatment.

CASE STUDY 2: PAEDIATRIC INTENSIVE CARE

Elaine Dhouieb

You are called to a 9-year-old girl on PICU with asthma, admitted with respiratory distress.

Telephone history

- Upper respiratory tract infection for 2 days, increasing inhaler use
- Intubated, ventilated, sedated and paralysed, size 4.5 nasal ET tube

- On i.v. salbutamol, steroids and antibiotics
- Ventilation – pressure control 24/3; 18 breaths per minute; 60% O_2
- ABGs – pH 7.2, pCO_2 9.3 kPa (70 mmHg), pO_2 10 kPa (75 mmHg), BE +3
- Vital signs – HR 120, BP 140/70, SpO_2 92%, temperature 38.3°C
- Auscultation – mild wheeze, decreased air entry right lower zone, crackles throughout
- Patient supine, head slightly elevated
- Suction – thick mucopurulent secretions
- CXR – 2 hours ago, showing right lower lobe collapse, hyperinflated left lung and gas in stomach.

Questions

1. Is this an appropriate call out?
2. Analyse the ABG
3. What could your treatment be?
4. What other treatments might you consider?
5. What else could you consider with the nursing staff?

Answers

1. Yes – retained secretions and CXR changes, monitor wheeze.
2. ABG:
- Borderline hypoxic
- Partially compensated respiratory acidosis.
3. Potential treatments:
- Left side-lying, flat or head up
- MHI – low PEEP (minimize air trapping)
- Slow percussion and vibrations (monitor wheeze)
- Saline (?warmed)
- Suction (+/– vibrations)
- Titrate FiO_2 to keep SpO_2 above 93%.
4. Other treatment options:
- Bronchoalveolar lavage for acute lobar collapse – if wheeze allows
- Right side-lying and MHI with vibrations/holds to decrease hyperinflation in left lung (manual decompressions).
5. Consider:
- ?Nasogastric tube on free drainage allows gas to escape from stomach – will aid diaphragm excursion
- Optimize humidification and fluids – ?dehydrated.

20

CASE STUDY 3: MEDICAL UNIT
Elizabeth Thomas

History

Mrs B, a 58-year-old known COPD patient, admitted via A&E complaining of 1-week history of ↑SOB, cough productive of purulent sputum, two episodes of haemoptysis, and right-sided pleuritic chest pain. She was previously admitted 3 weeks earlier and discharged 5 days later following treatment for exacerbation of COPD.

Past medical history
● Severe COPD
● Osteoporosis.

Social history
● 80 pack year smoking history – stopped smoking 6 months ago.
● Lives with husband who works. Husband assists with activities of daily living. Daughter visits daily.
● Exercise tolerance – SOB mobilizing from room to room at home. Goes out in wheelchair.
● Bathroom and bedroom downstairs.

Drug history
● Salbutamol nebulizer
● Spiriva (tiotropium) inhaler
● Seretide (salmeterol) inhaler
● Alendronate
● Vitamin D
● Calcichew.

Call out

On call physiotherapist asked to review patient diagnosed with exacerbation of COPD and hospital-acquired pneumonia. Respiratory function and ABGs deteriorating. Productive of purulent sputum.

From the end of the bed
Airway
● Spontaneous ventilation, airway patent. Speaking in short sentences.

Breathing
- ↑WOB
- Respiratory pattern: paradoxical breathing, active expiration, accessory muscles active
- RR 32 b.p.m.
- Sats 97% on FiO_2 0.4 via Venturi mask
- Pleuritic pain on coughing.

Circulation
- BP 105/60
- HR 105, sinus rhythm
- Temperature 38.2°C.

Current medical management
- i.v. antibiotics
- i.v. fluids
- 30 mg prednisolone
- Salbutamol and Atrovent (ipratropium) nebulizers
- FiO_2 0.4
- Alendronate
- Calcichew
- Vitamin D.

Investigations

CXR

Hyperinflated thorax, emphysematous bullae upper zones, shadowing and air bronchograms consistent with consolidation in right lower zone. Loss of medial half of right hemidiaphragm (silhouette sign).

CTPA (CT of pulmonary artery)
- Normal.

ABGs (on FiO_2 0.4)
- pH 7.30
- pO_2 11.4 kPa
- pCO_2 8.6 kPa
- HCO_3 34 mmol/L
- BE −4.4.

Bloods
- Hb 16.5 g/100 ml
- WBC 20×10^9/L
- Urea 12 mmol/L
- Creatinine 80 µmol/L.

Physical examination
Palpation
- Poor lower thoracic expansion (right = left) and ↑upper thoracic movement consistent with hyperinflation.

Auscultation
- BS quiet throughout with expiratory wheeze.
- Further ↓BS, right lower zone.
- Late inspiratory crackles, right lower zone.
- Early expiratory crackles transmitting from upper airways.

Percussion note
- Dull right lower zone
- Hyper-resonant elsewhere.

Questions
1. What do you need to consider prior to treating this patient, based on assessment findings?
2. What are your treatment options?

Answers
1. The following factors need to be considered:

Type II respiratory failure
Is the FiO_2 appropriate? The high Hb is indicative of chronically low pO_2 (polycythaemia) and raised bicarbonate suggests chronically high pCO_2 (chronic type II respiratory failure). This patient is likely to be oxygen sensitive and may have oxygen-induced respiratory acidosis. A target pO_2 of 8 kPa is probably more realistic for this patient.

Pain
Ensure adequate analgesia prior to treatment.

Haemoptysis

- When was the last episode of haemoptysis?
- Were there streaks of blood (commonly associated with pneumonia) or was it frank haemoptysis? How will this affect your choice of treatment?
- Note that PE has been ruled out by normal CTPA.
- Is the patient being investigated for cancer of the lung?
- You may want to check Hb levels.

Dehydration

The patient is dehydrated – raised urea with normal creatinine, low BP and ↑HR. This will hinder sputum clearance.

Osteoporosis

- Check CXR for fractures.
- Care with manual techniques.

Emphysematous bullae

There is an increased risk of pneumothorax with any positive pressure techniques in patients with bullous emphysema.

2. Treatment options:

- Liaise with medical staff regarding O_2 therapy (see above). If patient is still in type II respiratory failure following controlled O_2 therapy to achieve a more realistic pO_2, consider NIV. NB: There is a risk of pneumothorax with positive pressure treatments in patients with emphysematous bullae.
- Humidify O_2, encourage oral fluids, consider saline nebulizers ± mucolytics to assist with sputum clearance.
- Increase emphasis on breathing control in positions of ease during ACBT.
- If using manual techniques, reassess regularly to check that bronchospasm is not worsening, and use extra caution due to osteoporosis. Stop manual treatments if haemoptysis returns.
- Use positioning to reduce WOB and optimize V/Q matching. Modified positions may be required due to breathlessness.

CASE STUDY 4: SURGICAL UNIT

Valerie Ball

History

62-year-old male with a history of colonic cancer, had an elective right hemico-lectomy via a laparotomy incision 2 days ago. Seen by physiotherapist on first postoperative day when chest was noted to be clear, but he has become increasingly SOBAR since.

Past medical history

Normally fit and well. Ca colon diagnosed after patient noted change in bowel habit.

Social history

Retired company director, lives with wife, has three adult children; ex-smoker (25 pack year history, gave up 10 years ago), plays golf several times a week.

Call out

On call physio asked to review. Patient unable to expectorate and has an increasing respiratory rate which suggest postoperative chest infection.

From the end of the bed

Airway

- SOBAR, able to speak short sentences.

Breathing

- RR 28, saturating at 94% on 8 litres via simple low-flow face mask.

Circulation

- BP 162/85. Temp. 38.8°C. Pulse 112 b.p.m.
- NBM, i.v. fluid 100 ml/h.

Drug history

- Normally nil
- Since theatre:
  - PCA morphine – not being used at regular intervals
  - Stemetil (prochlorperazine) i.v. – for nausea
  - Clexane (enoxaparin sodium) s.c. injection – anticoagulant.

Investigations

- ECG sinus tachycardia
- ABGs:
  - pH 7.39
  - pCO_2 4.80

- pO_2 9.9
- HCO_3 23.1
- BE −1.0
- CXR Poor inspiratory volume and likely R > L bibasal atelectasis
- Blood counts:
  - Hb 11.6
  - WCC 13.2.

Physical examination

Palpation

Apical breathing, tactile fremitus over right mid-zone anteriorly.

Auscultation

Quiet BS throughout especially at bases, few crackles in URT.

Questions

1. What are the key elements of your assessment and why?
2. At this stage what are your treatment options?

Answers

1. Key assessment elements include the following:

General

- The patient was previously fit and well, but his past smoking history may have resulted in some residual mild COPD.

CVS

- Look at the HR and BP – these figures could suggest inadequate pain relief and/or infection.
- Raised WCC could indicate infection.

Respiratory

- He is not expanding his lungs effectively (CXR and auscultation).
- Atelectasis combined with infection would result in collapse/consolidation; volume loss would result in falling oxygen saturations.
- Palpation and auscultation also suggest some retained secretions.
- The oxygen is being delivered by a dry system; this could contribute to a retention problem and increase WOB.

20

2. Treatment options:

Analgesia
- Discuss with staff strategies to improve analgesia. Consider requesting a continuous i.v. morphine infusion or, if patient is capable, instruct in more effective use of PCA.
- Reassure patient that you do not wish to increase his pain.

Respiratory
- Initiate humidified oxygen through high-flow device with accurate % oxygen delivery. Start at 40% oxygen and monitor saturations and RR. Find admission saturation level in view of possible COPD – you may have to accept a lower than normal value.
- You may wish to give saline via nebulizer while humidify equipment warms up.
- Position in high side-lying to promote basal expansion.
- Teach (or revisit if previously taught) ACBT with wound support for coughing.

CASE STUDY 5: NEUROLOGICAL UNIT

Lorraine Clapham

Call to see a 52-year-old man admitted with progressive muscle weakness affecting all four limbs.

History
- PMH: No previous hospital admissions, minor illnesses only
- SH: Married, schoolteacher. Non-smoker; usually very active.

Medical findings on admission
- Alert, oriented
- Cranial nerves – intact
- Motor power – proximal muscle weakness grades 3–4
- Sensation – intact.

Respiratory system
- Trachea central, respiratory rate 20
- Normal breath sounds
- Vital capacity 5 litres
- CXR – elevated right hemidiaphragm

- ABGs:
  - pH 7.4, $PaCO_2$ 4.49, PaO_2 9.9
  - HCO_3 22
  - O_2 saturation 95% on air.

Provisional diagnosis
Guillain–Barré syndrome.

Call for physiotherapy
6 hours after admission.

Reason given for call out
Vital capacity has fallen to 1.6 litres; now requiring 35% oxygen and is maintaining oxygen saturation levels at 96%.

Questions
1. Given that oxygen saturation levels are being maintained at 96% on FiO_2 of 35%, from the information provided what indications are there for emergency on call physiotherapy?
2. What further information will you require, and what will be the key elements of your assessment?
3. At this stage, what are your treatment options (management plan)?

Answers
1. Indications for emergency physiotherapy:
- There has been a rapid and major deterioration in the patient's condition. Vital capacity has fallen by 68% from 5 litres to 1.6 litres. The patient's ability to take a sigh breath is impaired, as is their ability to clear any retained secretions. Some degree of atelectasis will have already occurred. This will probably progress to major lobar collapse and sputum retention.
- On admission there were already signs that would have predicted the possibility of respiratory deterioration:
  a. The elevated right diaphragm in the absence of obvious lobar collapse suggests that there is some degree of paralysis of this muscle.
  b. The high respiratory rate and low CO_2 suggest that the patient is working very hard to maintain his PaO_2 and oxygen saturation levels at 96%.
- Without intervention this patient is likely to fatigue quickly and progress to respiratory failure and require ventilation.

20

2. Further information required:
● Observe and assess the patient.
● Arterial blood gases are essential; the patient may already be retaining CO_2.
● Repeat chest X-ray.
● Is there any indication that the patient may be at risk of aspiration, e.g. wet-sounding voice, reports of coughing when drinking?

3. Treatment options:
● Position the patient so as to reduce the work of breathing (see Chapter 8).
● Humidify oxygen.
● Reassure the patient.
● IPPB to inflate lung and improve lung compliance thus reducing the work of breathing and oxygen demand.
● Patient review in 1 h; repeat vital capacity and ABGs.
● If CO_2 continues to rise ventilation will need to be discussed. Depending on the team decision this may be NIV, if available, or full ventilation. Care must be taken not to mask a deteriorating patient – close monitoring is essential.
● Review as planned.
● Inform staff of current action plan and leave contact number.
● If patient's condition stabilizes or improves, continue with current treatment plan and monitoring.
● Ensure the ICU has been alerted to the problem. If the patient continues to deteriorate, a planned intubation is preferable to an emergency intubation.

CASE STUDY 6: CARDIOTHORACIC UNIT

Angela Kell

A 55-year-old man, post CABG × 3 yesterday. Initially progressed well and was out of bed this morning; however during the course of the evening has become more breathless, hypoxic and anxious. He is a lifelong non-smoker.

On arrival

● Patient has PCA morphine but is very tense and complaining of pain
● Obese gentleman, slumped in bed
● BP 100/60, HR 110 ST, CVP 12
● Bloods – WCC 14.5, Hb 10, CRP 150, albumin 24
● UO 20 ml per hour, last 3 hours. Fluid balance positive 2 litres
● Self-ventilating on FiO_2 98% via face mask (humidified), RR 25 (laboured), SpO_2 92%. On auscultation: barely audible breath sounds basally with a few late inspiratory crackles. Equal but poor chest expansion

- ABGs – pH 7.37, pO_2 8.2 kPa, pCO_2 4.5 kPa, HCO_3 22, BE 1
- CXR – awaited.

Questions

1. a. What are his main physio problems?
   b. What are his main medical problems?
2. What might prevent you from mobilizing this patient?
3. What treatment options are available to you?
4. What would you like to discuss with his doctors?
5. What objective markers could you use to assess change?

Answers

1. a. Pain, bibasal collapse, increased work of breathing, reduced expansion, anxiety, hypoxia.
   b. Inadequate pain control, hypotension (likely causing poor renal function), pulmonary oedema, potential infection brewing.
2. Minimal respiratory reserve, hypotension (likely to worsen when upright), pain and anxiety (will heighten respiratory demand).
3. Reassure and reposition; if upright sitting, ensure abdomen does not impinge on diaphragmatic excursion. CPAP – check CXR first. Remember his size: he will need big PEEP (10 cmH_2O) and a high flow to meet his inspiratory flow demand. Will also need a high FiO_2 until an improvement in ABGs is evident.
4. Optimization of analgesia and review of poor urine output. Discuss use of CPAP and possible movement to a higher level of care.
5. Auscultation, ABGs, FiO_2, SpO_2, RR and WOB.

CASE STUDY 7: THORACIC UNIT

Angela Kell

45-year-old woman, had a left lower lobectomy 2 days ago. She has good pain control via an epidural, but is unable to clear sputum. She gave up heavy smoking 8 weeks ago.

On arrival

- Patient sat in chair.
- BP 110/75, HR 80 SR, adequate urine output, fluid balance positive 500 ml.
- Self ventilating on 4 litres O_2 via nasal prongs, SpO_2 94%, RR 18 normal pattern, cough wet and weak. Palpable fremitus on anterior chest wall and poor expansion on left. Auscultation: widespread transmitted coarse expiratory crackles, with reduced breath sounds left lower zone. Two chest drains in situ (one apical, one basal). Apical chest drain is bubbling – both drains on suction.

Questions

1. Why is the apical chest drain bubbling?
2. What are her main problems?
3. What are your treatment options?

Answers

1. Failure of the pleura to stick up postoperatively due to a persistent air leak from the lung into the intrapleural space.
2. Sputum retention, poor tidal volume.
3. Mobilize (check chest drains can come off suction) – to increase her tidal volumes. If she is on strict suction, march on spot, or use exercise bike (if available). Supported coughing/huffing should aid sputum clearance. Consider nebulizers (saline or salbutamol) for really sticky sputum and consider changing to humidified oxygen therapy.

CASE STUDY 8: HAEMATOLOGY PATIENT

Irelna Kruger and Katharine Malhotra

Background

65-year-old male with a long history of chronic lymphocytic leukaemia (CLL), had donor bone marrow transplant 3 months ago. Admitted yesterday generally unwell with a 3–4-day history of persistent dry cough and SOBOE. Asked to review as deteriorating respiratory function with CXR changes. Doctors requesting sputum specimen.

Past medical history

10 years ago CLL – had an autograft (own bone marrow transplant) with chemotherapy and total body irradiation (TBI).

Social history

Lives with wife, two adult children, lifelong non-smoker.

On arrival

- A – SOBAR, unable to speak full sentences
- B – RR 32, SpO$_2$ 92% on 60% O$_2$ via face mask
- C – BP 95/60; Temp. 38.5; Pulse 126 b.p.m. (sinus tachycardia)
- Fluids in progress.

Drug history

- Immunosuppressants.

Investigations

- ABGs:
  - pH 7.24
  - pCO_2 4.80
  - PO_2 11.4
  - HCO_3 14.9
  - BE −11.0
- CXR shows bibasal consolidation
- Blood counts Hb 9.3, WCC 0.2, Plts 22.

Auscultation/palpation

- Harsh BS throughout with bibasal crackles
- Apical expansion only.

Questions

1. What are the key elements of your assessment and why?
2. What are your treatment options?

Answers

1. Key assessment elements include the following:

General

- Due to long treatment history, consider fatigue and nutritional status.

CVS

- Note tachycardia with a low BP and pyrexia. This patient is exhibiting signs of sepsis (be aware, immunosuppressants may mask signs of infection as they keep WCC low).
- Review blood counts and be aware of the implications of low platelets. A low WCC may result in low sputum production (atypical infection).

Respiratory

- Previous TBI may cause fibrotic changes to lungs.
- ABGs: is patient compensating for a metabolic acidosis with an increased respiratory rate?

2. Treatment options:
- Recognize extreme limitations due to cardiovascular instability.
- You could position to reduce WOB, and CPAP may be appropriate. However, this patient needs senior medical review and potentially more invasive support.

CASE STUDY 9: ONCOLOGY PATIENT

Irelna Kruger and Katharine Malhotra

History

Called to a 73-year-old female with previous squamous cell carcinoma (SCC) of oesophagus. 3 weeks post-oesophageal bypass procedure and feeding jejunostomy for radiotherapy-induced oesophageal stricture. Postoperative recovery complicated by left vocal cord palsy. Currently suspected aspiration causing respiratory distress. Although speech and language therapist recommended NBM, specialist registrar deemed patient safe for soft diet.

Past medical history

- SCC oesophagus diagnosed 6 years previously, treated with chemotherapy and radiotherapy.
- Breast cancer 25 years ago, known single pulmonary metastasis.

Social history

- Widow, lives with son.
- Ex-smoker.

On arrival

A – SOB, 'wet' incoherent voice

B – RR 22, SpO_2 84% on 98% humidified O_2 via face mask

C – BP 151/70; Temp. 36.3°C; Pulse 102 b.p.m. (sinus tachycardia).

Drug history

- Tamoxifen.

Investigations

- ABGs:
  - pH 7.42
  - pCO_2 6.38
  - pO_2 8.32
  - HCO_3 29.8
  - BE 6.5
- CXR shows right middle lobe patchy shadowing
- Blood counts: Hb 9.5, WCC 17.0, Platelets 185, CRP 284.

Auscultation/palpation

- Widespread coarse crackles with tactile fremitus.

Questions

1. What are the key elements of your assessment and why?
2. What are your treatment options?

Answers

1. Key assessment elements include the following:

General
● Sudden deterioration
● Recent oesophageal surgery – note altered anatomy and contraindications/ cautions to treatment
● Long history of swallowing difficulties.

CVS
● Signs of infection – tachycardia with raised WCC and CRP.

CNS
● Signs of confusion, could be due to:
  ○ hypoxia
  ○ neurological event
  ○ brain metastases.

Respiratory
● Single pulmonary metastasis (be aware of).

2. Treatment options:
● Ascertain if appropriate for critical care and resus status. She is acutely unwell and needs immediate action to avoid further deterioration.
● Liaise with medical team regarding suction and IPPB. Needs to be documented before undertaking these treatments due to altered anatomy and risk of damage to anastomosis.
● May be too fatigued and confused for ACBT and has an ineffective cough due to vocal cord palsy. Therefore positioning, manual techniques and suction (if team consent) may be only options.

CASE STUDY 10: PAEDIATRIC WARD
Paul Ritson

You are called to see a 5-year-old girl with cerebral palsy on the paediatric ward. Admitted with increased seizures.

Telephone history
- Severe developmental delay and spasticity
- Possible aspiration 1 hour ago
- SpO$_2$ 88% in 15 litres oxygen via mask
- Suction – copious thick green secretions
- ABGs: pH 7.25, pCO$_2$ 10 kPa (75 mmHg), pO$_2$ 8 kPa (60 mmHg), BE +1
- Recent CXR (Fig. 20.1) – not reported
- Auscultation: Reduced breath sounds bibasally, crackles right > left.

Questions
1. What further information do you require? Can you offer any advice?
2. How would you plan your assessment?
3. Analyse ABGs and CXR.
4. Devise a treatment plan; justify your answers.

Answers
1. Further information required:
- Response to handling
- Position of patient
- Clinical details, e.g. CVS

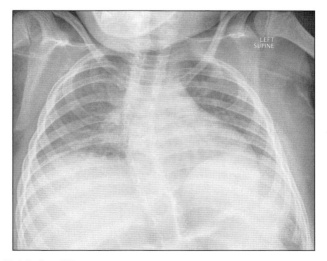

Figure 20.1 Patient CXR.

- Suction frequency/type (NP/OP)
- Nebulizers. Which ones?
- Relevant PMH.

Advice:
- Increase FiO_2, keeping SpO_2 above 93%, humidify via face mask
- Reposition to supported side-lying with 'head up'
- Bronchodilator (if prescribed)/saline nebulizer.

2. Assessment:
- ABC (see Chapter 4).

3. Interpretation:
CXR:
- Thoracic scoliosis
- Small volume lungs
- No major consolidation/collapse
- Mild right lower zone changes, ?infection.
ABG:
- Hypoxic
- Uncompensated respiratory acidosis.

4. Treatment plan:
- Consent!
- Maximize oxygen therapy – keep SpO_2 >93%
- Humidification
- ?Saline/bronchodilator nebulizers
- Positioning (alternate side-lying, head up), modify if desaturates
- ?Manual techniques
- ?NP suction
- Regular repositioning/reassessment
- **Never treat when fitting**
- **Communication with parents/team.**

Abbreviations

A&E: Accident & Emergency

ABC: Airway, Breathing, Circulation

ABG: arterial blood gas

ACBT: active cycle of breathing techniques

ACE: angiotensin converting enzyme

ACPRC: Association of Chartered Physiotherapists in Respiratory Care

AD: autogenic drainage

AF: atrial fibrillation

ALI: acute lung injury

AML: acute myeloid leukaemia

AP: anteroposterior

APTT: activated partial thromboplastin time

ARDS: acute respiratory distress syndrome

ASAP: as soon as possible

ASB: assisted spontaneous breathing

ASD: atrial septal defect

Ausc.: auscultation

AV: arterioventricular

AVPU: best patient response, **A**lert, responding to **V**oice, **P**ain or is **U**nresponsive

AVSD: atrioventricular septal defect

AVR: aortic valve replacement

BAL: bronchoalveolar lavage

BC: breathing control

BE: base excess

BiPAP: bi-level positive airway pressure

BMI: body mass index

BOS: base of skull

BP: blood pressure (arterial)

b.p.m./BPM: beats per minute (also used as breaths per minute)

BPD: bronchopulmonary dysplasia

b.p.m.: beats per minute

BS: breath sounds

BTS: British Thoracic Society

Ca: cancer

CABG: coronary artery bypass graft

CCF: congestive cardiac failure

CF: cystic fibrosis

CFM: cerebral function monitor

CMD: congenital muscular dystrophy

CMV: continuous mandatory ventilation

CMV: cytomegalovirus

CNS: central nervous system

CO_2: carbon dioxide

COAD: chronic obstructive airway disease

COPD: chronic obstructive pulmonary disease

CP: cerebral palsy

CPD: continuing professional development

CPAP: continuous positive airway pressure

CPP: cerebral perfusion pressure

CRP: C-reactive protein

CRT: capillary refill time

CSF: cerebrospinal fluid

CSP: Chartered Society of Physiotherapy

CT: computed tomography

CVA: cerebrovascular accident

CVVHD: continuous veno-venous haemodialysis

CVVHF: continuous veno-venous haemofiltration

CVP: central venous pressure

CVS: cardiovascular system

CXR: chest X-ray

DH: drug history

DIC: disseminated intravascular coagulation

DMD: Duchenne muscular dystrophy

DVT: deep vein thrombosis

ECG: electrocardiogram

ECMO: extracorporeal membrane oxygenation

ENT: Ear Nose & Throat

EPAP: expiratory positive airway pressure

ET: endotracheal

ETT: endotracheal tube

EVD: external ventricular drain

Fen.: fenestrated

FET: forced expiration technique

FEV_1: forced vital capacity in first second of expiration

FiO_2: fraction of inspired oxygen

FRC: functional residual capacity

FVC: forced vital capacity

GAP: gravity-assisted positioning

GCS: Glasgow Coma Scale

GI: gastrointestinal

GOR: gastro-oesophageal reflux

GTN: glyceryl trinitrate

Hb: haemoglobin

HCO_3: bicarbonate

HDU: high dependency unit

HF: haemofiltration

HFO: high-frequency oscillation

HFOV: high-frequency oscillatory ventilation

HME: heat and moisture exchanger

HPC: history of present condition

HR: heart rate

IABP: intra-aortic balloon pump

ICD: intercostal drain

ICP: intracranial pressure

ICU: intensive care unit

IHD: ischaemic heart disease

i.m.: intramuscular

INR: international normalized ratio

IPPB: intermittent positive pressure breathing

IPPV: intermittent positive pressure ventilation

IS: incentive spirometry

i.v.: intravenous

JVP: jugular venous pressure

K^+: potassium ions

LFT: lung function test *or* liver function test

LLL: left lower lobe

LPA: lasting power of attorney

LTEE: lower thoracic expansion exercise

LTOT: long-term oxygen therapy

LUL: left upper lobe

LVF: left ventricular failure

LZ: lower zone

MAP: mean arterial pressure

MDT: multidisciplinary team

MEWS: Modified Early Warning Score

MHI: manual hyperinflation

MI: myocardial infarction

MT: manual techniques

MRSA: methicillin-resistant *Staphylococcus aureus*

MV: minute volume

MVR: mitral valve replacement

MZ: middle zone

Na^+: sodium ions

NaCl: sodium chloride

NAI: non-accidental injury

NBM: nil by mouth

NCA: nurse-controlled analgesia

NEC: necrotizing enterocolitis

NGT: nasogastric tube

NIV: non-invasive ventilation

NO: nitric oxide

NP: nasopharyngeal

NSAIDs: non-steroidal anti-inflammatory drugs

O_2: oxygen

OP: oropharyngeal

PA: pulmonary artery

PA: posteroanterior

$PaCO_2$: partial pressure of carbon dioxide in arterial blood

PaO_2: partial pressure of oxygen in arterial blood

PAP: peak airway pressure

PAWP: pulmonary artery wedge pressure

PCA: patient-controlled analgesia

PCEA: patient-controlled epidural anaesthesia/analgesia

PCP: *Pneumocystis carinii* pneumonia

PCPAP: periodic CPAP

PD: postural drainage

PDP: personal development plan

PE: pulmonary embolus

PEEP: positive end expiratory pressure

PEFR: peak expiratory flow rate

PEP: positive expiratory pressure

pH: negative logarithm of hydrogen ion concentration in moles per litre

PICC: peripherally inserted central catheter

PICU: paediatric intensive care unit

PIP: positive inspiratory pressure

Plts: platelets

PMH: past medical history

p.r.n.: 'as required'

PRVC: pressure-regulated volume control

PS: pressure support *or* pulmonary stenosis

PT: prothrombin time

PVC: premature ventricular contraction

PVD: peripheral vascular disease

RLL: right lower lobe

RML: right middle lobe

RR: respiratory rate

RS: respiratory system

RSV: respiratory syncytial virus

RTA: road traffic accident

RUL: right upper lobe

SAH: subarachnoid haemorrhage

SaO_2: saturation of oxygen in arterial blood (shown in ABGs)

SB: spina bifida

s.c.: subcutaneous

SNP: sodium nitroprusside

SH: social history

SIRS: systemic inflammatory response syndrome

SMA: spinal muscular atrophy

SR: sinus rhythm

SSC: squamous cell carcinoma

ST: sinus tachycardia

SOB: shortness of breath

SOBAR: shortness of breath at rest

SOBOE: shortness of breath on exertion

A1

SpO$_2$: pulse oximetry arterial oxygen saturation
SVCO: superior vena cava obstruction
SWOT: strengths, weaknesses, opportunities, threats
TB: tuberculosis
TBI: total body irradiation
TEE: thoracic expansion exercise
TENS: transcutaneous electrical nerve stimulation
TGA: transposition of great arteries
TMR: transmyocardial revascularization

TOF: tetralogy of Fallot
TV: tidal volume
UO: urinary output
URT: upper respiratory tract
UZ: upper zone
V$_T$: tidal volume
VAS: visual analogue scale
V/Q: ventilation/perfusion ratio
VC: vital capacity
VSD: ventricular septal defect
WCC: white cell count
WOB: work of breathing

Normal values

Table to show normal values. Reproduced from Pryor and Prasad (2008), with permission.

Normal values for arterial blood gases
pH: 7.35–7.45
PaO_2: 10.7–13.3 kPa (80–100 mmHg)
$PaCO_2$: 4.7–6.0 kPa (35–45 mmHg)
HCO_3: 22–26 mmol/L
Base excess: −2 to +2
From Pryor JA, Prasad SA (eds) (2008) Physiotherapy for respiratory and cardiac problems, 4th edn. London: Churchill Livingstone (Box 1.4).

Normal values for blood pressure (BP) (adult)

Normal value of systolic/diastolic pressure: 95/60 − 140/90 mmHg

Normal value of mean arterial pressure = Diastolic + [(Systolic − Diastolic)/3] = 70–110 mmHg

From Pryor JA, Prasad SA (eds) (2008) Physiotherapy for respiratory and cardiac problems, 4th edn. London: Churchill Livingstone (Box 8.2).

Normal values for central venous pressure (CVP)

Normal CVP: 3–15 cmH_2O (2.2–11 mmHg)

From Pryor JA, Prasad SA (eds) (2008) Physiotherapy for respiratory and cardiac problems, 4th edn. London: Churchill Livingstone (Box 8.3).

A2

Paediatric normal values

	Newborn	Up to 3 years	3–6 years	>6 years
Arterial blood pH	7.30–7.40	7.30–7.40	7.35–7.45	7.35–7.45
$PaCO_2$ (mmHg) (kPa)	30–35 4.0–4.7	30–35 4.0–4.7	35–45 4.7–6.0	35–45 4.7–6.0
PaO_2 (mmHg) (kPa)	60–90 8.0–12.0	80–100 10.7–13.3	80–100 10.7–13.3	80–100 10.7–13.3

Adapted from Pryor JA, Prasad SA (eds) (2008) Physiotherapy for respiratory and cardiac problems, 4th edn. London: Churchill Livingstone (Table 9.5).

Paediatric normal values

Age group	Heart rate – mean (range) (beats/min)	Respiratory rate – range (breaths/min)	Blood pressure – systolic/diastolic (mmHg)
Preterm	150 (100–200)	40–60	39–59/16–36
Newborn	140 (80–200)	30–50	50–70/25–45
<2 years	130 (100–190)	20–40	87–105/53–66
>2 years	80 (60–140)	20–40	95–105/53–66
>6 years	75 (60–90)	15–30	97–112/57–71

From Pryor JA, Prasad SA (eds) (2008) Physiotherapy for respiratory and cardiac problems, 4th edn. London: Churchill Livingstone (Table 13.1).

Conversion tables

| 0.133 kPa = 5 1.0 mmHg | | pH = 9 − log [H⁺] where [H⁺] is in nmol/L | |
kPa	mmHg	pH	[H⁺]
1	7.5	7.52	30
2	15.0	7.45	35
4	30	7.40	40
6	45	7.35	45
8	60	7.30	50
10	75	7.26	55
12	90	7.22	60
14	105	7.19	65

From Pryor JA, Prasad SA (eds) (2002) Physiotherapy for respiratory and cardiac problems, 3rd edn. London: Churchill Livingstone.

BLOOD CHEMISTRY

Albumin	37–53 g/L
Calcium (Ca^{2+})	2.25–2.65 mmol/L
Creatinine	60–120 µmol/L
Glucose	4–6 mmol/L
Potassium (K^+)	3.4–5.0 mmol/L
Sodium (Na^+)	134–140 mmol/L
Urea	2.5–6.5 mmol/L
Haemoglobin (Hb)	14.0–18.0 g/100 ml (men) 11.5–15.5 g/100 ml (women)
Platelets	$150–400 \times 10^9$/L
White blood cell count (WCC)	$4–11 \times 10^9$/L
Urine output	1 ml/kg/h

From Pryor JA, Prasad SA (eds) (2002) Physiotherapy for respiratory and cardiac problems, 3rd edn. London: Churchill Livingstone.

Surgical incisions

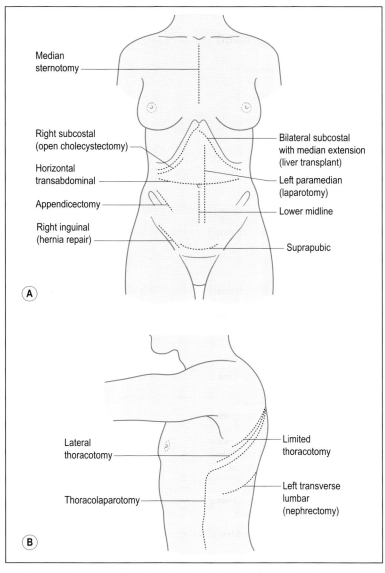

Figure showing common surgical incisions. Reproduced from Pryor and Prasad (2002), with kind permission.

Common drugs used in critical care areas

Angela Kell

Group	Effect	Indications	Examples
Bronchodilators	Relax smooth muscles of the airways	Bronchospasm	Salbutamol (Ventolin) Bricanyl Atrovent
Mucolytics	Reduce the viscosity of sputum to aid airway clearance	Viscous sputum	N-acetyl-cysteine (Parvolex) Carbocisteine (Mucodyne) Hypertonic saline DNase (Pulmozyme)
Inotropes	Increase the force of myocardial contraction increasing cardiac output Relax smooth muscle, increasing preload and afterload	Heart failure	Enoximone Milrinone
Glycosides	Slow electrical conduction through the AV node	Heart failure Supraventricular tachycardias	Digoxin
Diuretics	Promote excretion of water and electrolytes by the renal system		
Thiazides	Inhibit sodium reabsorption	Chronic heart failure Hypertension (low doses only)	Bendroflumethiazide Indapamide Metolazone

A4

Group	Effect	Indications	Examples
Loop diuretics	Inhibit fluid reabsorption in the renal tubule	Pulmonary oedema and left ventricular failure. They are the most powerful diuretics	Furosemide (frusemide) Bumetanide Lasix
Potassium sparing diuretics	Increase water and electrolyte excretion but prevent loss of potassium and hydrogen ions	Diuretic-induced hypokalaemia. Oedema due to chronic heart failure. Hypertension	Amiloride Spironolactone Co-amilofruse
Sympathomimetics	Mimic sympathetic nervous system – constrict peripheral blood vessels, increase heart rate	Hypotension	Dobutamine Dopamine Noradrenaline Epinephrine Norepinephrine
Anti-arrhythmics	Different drugs will target different arrhythmias by either sodium channel blocking, beta-adrenergic receptor blocking or calcium channel blocking	Ventricular tachycardias, atrial flutter and fibrillation, paroxysmal tachycardias, supraventricular tachycardias, ventricular fibrillation	Amiodarone Diltiazem Verapamil Adenosine Flecainide Sotalol Quinidine
Nitrates	Coronary dilatation. Reduces venous return which reduces left ventricular workload	Acute angina relief	Isosorbide mononitrate (ISMN) Isosorbide dinitrate Glyceryl trinitrate (GTN)
Beta-blockers	Reduce blood pressure and slow heart rate, reducing the force of myocardial contraction, thus reducing myocardial oxygen demand	Hypertension. Long-term prevention of angina	Propranolol Atenolol Bisoprolol Metoprolol Labetalol

Group	Effect	Indications	Examples
Calcium channel blockers	Dilate coronary arteries by inhibiting calcium ion channels across the cell membrane, reducing the force of contraction and thus workload of the heart	Angina Some calcium channel blockers also have anti-arrhythmic properties	Diltiazem Nifedipine Amlodipine Felodipine
Antihypertensives	Work by inhibiting the sympathetic nervous system which dilates peripheral blood vessels, by blocking the calcium channels or by acting directly to dilate vessels	Hypertension First treatment of choice is beta-blockers and diuretics, followed by sympatholytics, vasodilators and ACE inhibitors SNP and GTN may be administered i.v. postoperatively to prevent spasm of grafted arteries, ensuring adequate myocardial perfusion	Sodium nitroprusside (SNP) See also beta-blockers, ACE inhibitors and diuretics
ACE inhibitors	Promote excretion of sodium and water; this lowers BP by decreasing cardiac output	Heart failure Hypertension Prophylaxis of cardiovascular events	Ramipril Lisinopril Captopril Enalapril
Statins	Inhibit enzymes involved in cholesterol synthesis, reducing arterial lipid deposition	Hypercholesterolaemia Secondary prevention of coronary and cardiovascular events	Atorvastatin Simvastatin
Potassium channel activators	Activate potassium channels, vasodilate vessels	Prophylaxis and treatment of angina	Nicorandil

A4

A4

Group	Effect	Indications	Examples
Anticoagulants	Reduce the ability of the blood to clot	DVT and PE prevention and treatment Prophylaxis for mechanical valve patients DIC	Heparin Enoxaparin Aspirin Warfarin
Thrombolytics	Dissolve pre-existing clots	PE DVT MI Ischaemic stroke	Streptokinase
Sedatives and anaesthetic agents	Depress CNS activity	For intubated/ ventilated patients	Propofol Midazolam Fentanyl
Analgesics	Depress pain pathways Can be opiate based or non-opiate based	Routinely administered after surgery – initially should be intravenous, via epidural or intramuscular, then progressed to oral where appropriate	Alfentanil Morphine Tramadol Paracetamol
Paralysing agents	Relaxation of respiratory and skeletal muscles	Due to difficulties in achieving optimal ventilation or to control neurological parameters, e.g. acute head injury	Atracurium Vecuronium Pancuronium
Anti-emetics	Block receptors in the GI tract and CNS	Nausea and vomiting (often induced by anaesthesia and analgesics). Often used prophylactically	Cyclizine Granisetron Ondansetron
Insulin	Regulates protein, fat and carbohydrate metabolism	Unstable/abnormal blood sugar levels Proven to improve wound healing in post-surgical population	Actrapid

A

ABC (Airway, Breathing, Circulation) assessment 17–18

abdominal breathing technique 237, 238, 239

abdominal surgery patient 162–4

Acapella device 240–1

active cycle of breathing techniques (ACBT) 237–40

acute cardiology patient 202–3

acute epiglottitis, children 48

acute lobar pneumonia, hypoxaemia 114

acute lung injury see ALI

acute respiratory distress syndrome see ARDS 131

acute respiratory failure see respiratory failure

adjuncts for respiratory physiotherapy treatments 240–1

adult intensive care unit (ICU) calls 123–35

alarm systems in the ICU 127–30

assessment of the ICU patient 123–5

bronchospasm 134

case study 273–4

common pathologies and conditions 131–3

drugs encountered in intensive care 131

environment of the ICU 125–30

equipment in the ICU 125–30

fatigue 134

identifying the cause of an alarm 127–30

lobar collapse 134

location of critically ill patients 123

management of ICU problems 134

pleural effusion 134

pneumothorax 134

pulmonary embolus 134

pulmonary oedema 134

sputum retention 134

Adults with Incapacity (Scotland) Act (2000) 15

advance decision (under the Mental Capacity Act 2005) 15

air bronchogram, chest X-ray interpretation 60, 61

airway differences in children 40, 41

airway resistance, effects of decreased FRC 87–8

ALI (acute lung injury) 131

lung volume loss 92, 96

alveolar pulmonary oedema, chest X-ray interpretation 59, 61, 64–5

alveolar ventilation, consequences of decreased V_T 89

anaemic hypoxaemia 112

aortic aneurysm 165

ARDS (acute respiratory distress syndrome) 131

complication of pancreatitis 150

lung volume loss 92, 96

arterial blood gas (ABG) tensions, in respiratory failure 111

arterial bypass graft 165

aspiration, chest X-ray interpretation 59, 60, 61

assisted cough 245–7

Association of Physiotherapists in Respiratory Care (ACPRC), assessment tool 1

asthma, acute 147–8

atelectasis/collapse

adult intensive care patient 134

chest X-ray interpretation 54–9, 63

lung volume loss 92, 97

auscultation

children 44, 47

patient assessment, 32–4

autogenic drainage 241

AVPU neurological assessment 24

axillo-femoral bypass 165

B

bagging technique 242–3

basal metabolic rate in infants 38

bradycardia response to hypoxia in children 38

brain-injured patient 178–83

breathing control technique 237–8, 239

bronchiectasis, medical unit calls 157

bronchiolitis, children 48

bronchopneumonia

hypoxaemia 114

medical unit calls 152, 154

bronchospasm

adult intensive care patient 134

and increased work of breathing 101, 103–4

sputum retention management 83

Burkholderia cepacia 156
burns, ICU calls 132–3

C

CABG (coronary artery bypass grafting) 190
cancer *see* oncology unit calls
capacity issues 14–16
Carbocisteine 109
carbon dioxide retention
   acute-on-chronic respiratory/ ventilatory failure 120
   causes of acute ventilatory failure 116–17
   causes of chronic ventilatory failure 119–20
   consequence of decreased V_T 89
   contraindication for CPAP 91
   hypoxaemia 115
   medications for chronic ventilatory failure 120
   signs and symptoms 113, 116
   treatment of hypercapnia 117–19
   see also hypercapnia
cardiac surgery patient 189–91, 192–3, 194–5
cardiology patient 202–3
cardiothoracic trauma patient 198, 200, 201–2
cardiothoracic unit calls 189–203
   cardiac surgery patient 189–91, 192–3, 194–5
   cardiology patient 202–3
   cardiothoracic trauma patient 198, 200, 201–2
   case study 284–5
   lung contusions 200, 201, 202
   rib fractures 198, 201, 202
   stab injuries 200, 201, 202
   thoracic surgery patient 191, 196–98, 199, 200–1
cardiovascular observations, patient assessment 22–3
case studies 273–91
   adult intensive care 273–4
   cardiothoracic unit 284–5
   haematology patient 286–7
   learning from on call events 5
   medical unit 276–9
   neurological unit 282–4
   oncology patient 288–9

paediatric intensive care 274–5
paediatric ward 289–91
surgical unit 279–82
thoracic unit 285–6
cerebral perfusion pressure (CPP) values 179, 181
Chartered Society of Physiotherapy, standards for on call working 1
chest X-ray interpretation 28–30
chest X-ray interpretation (abnormalities) 52–70
   air bronchogram 60, 61
   alveolar pulmonary oedema 59, 61, 64–5
   atelectasis/collapse 54–9, 63
   collapse/atelectasis 54–9, 63
   consolidation 59–63
   COPD (chronic obstructive pulmonary disease) 69
   emphysema 69
   fields which are too white 54–67
   fields which are too black 54, 66–9
   fluid in the lung 59–63
   heart failure and pulmonary oedema 64–5
   infected fluid in the lung 59, 63
   interstitial pulmonary oedema 66–7
   Kerley B lines 66, 67
   lobular collapse 54–7, 59
   loss of lung volume 54–9, 63
   lung collapse 54, 58–9
   pleural effusion 63–4, 65, 66
   pneumonectomy 54, 58
   pneumonia 59, 63
   pneumothorax 66–8, 69
   positioning of endotracheal tube 59
   pulmonary oedema 59, 61, 64–6, 67
   results of aspiration 59, 60, 61
   round pneumonia 63
   tension pneumothorax 66–8
   thoracotomy 54
   traumatic lung contusion 59, 60, 61–2
chest X-ray interpretation (normal) 51–2
   aortic arch 52
   costophrenic angle 52

factors affecting X-ray quality 51
heart shadow 52
hemidiaphragm (left and right) 52
hilum (left and right) 52
horizontal fissure 51, 52, 53
lingula 51
normal lobar anatomy 51–3
oblique fissure 51, 53
planes and zones of the lungs 52, 53
children *see* paediatric care
chronic chest disease, hypoxaemia 115
chronic obstructive pulmonary disease *see* COPD
clinical assessment *see* patient assessment
clinical experience, preparation for on call working 8–9
clinical reasoning process 5
clinicians, disagreement among 13–14
closing volume (lung) 85, 87
clotting disorders, ICU calls 133
collapse (lobar)
   adult intensive care patient 134
   lung volume loss 92, 97
collapse/atelectasis, chest X-ray interpretation 54–9, 63
communication
   disagreement among clinicians 13–14
   when to seek help 14
   with a child 38
   with parents 38
   with the medical/nursing staff 13
   with the patient/relatives 13
consent issues 14–16
   paediatric care 37
consolidation
   chest X-ray interpretation 59–63
   lung volume loss 92, 96
continuous positive airway pressure *see* CPAP
contractual issues, on call policy/procedures 8
COPD (chronic obstructive pulmonary disease)
   care of patient with end-stage COPD 146–7
   causes of hypoxaemia 145

causes of readmission 146, 147
chest X-ray interpretation 69
controlled oxygen therapy 145–6
hypoxic drive to stimulate breathing 146
increased work of breathing 109
medical unit calls 145–7
oxygen-induced respiratory acidosis 146
oxygen sensitive patients 146
risks of positive pressure ventilation 69
use of NIV in patients with respiratory acidosis 146
Cornet (R.C. Cornet®) device 240–1
coronary artery bypass grafting (CABG) 190
coronavirus 155
cough 244
assisted 245–7
ineffective 77, 78–9
cough assist device 247
cough stimulation/tracheal rub 248
CPAP (continuous positive airway pressure) 248–9
and carbon dioxide retention 91
contraindication in pneumothorax 67
risks with COPD 69
use in lung volume loss 91, 95–100
CPP (cerebral perfusion pressure) values 179, 181
critical care, location of patients 123 see also intensive care unit (ICU); paediatric intensive care unit (PICU)
critical incident report (learning context) 4, 5
croup (acute laryngotracheobronchitis), children 48
cyanosis, in children 44
cystic fibrosis
medical unit calls 153, 155–6
sputum retention 74

D

debrief after an on call event 3–4

deep breathing exercises 237, 238, 239
dehydration, and sputum retention 77, 82
diaphragmatic breathing 237–8, 239
documentation of on call events 16
drainage
gravity-assisted 258, 260–2
postural 258, 260–2

E

early warning scores, patient assessment 34–5
ECG monitoring, patient assessment 23–4
emphysema, chest X-ray interpretation 69
endotracheal suction 267–9
endotracheal tube positioning, chest X-ray interpretation 59
ENT surgery patient 167
Erdoseine 109
external fixators, surgical patients 166

F

facial/intra-oral reconstruction 168
fatigue
adult intensive care patient 134
hypoxaemic patients 115
feedback
to other professionals 16
to patient/relatives 16
femoro-popliteal bypass 165
flail chest, lung volume loss 93, 98
fluid in the lung, chest X-ray interpretation 59–63
Flutter device 240–1
forced expiration technique (FET) 237, 238, 239–40
forced vital capacity (FVC) 85, 86, 89–90
causes of decreased FVC 89
consequences of decreased FVC 90
functional residual capacity (FRC) 85–9, 95
causes of decreased FRC 85, 87
consequences of decreased FRC 87–9

fungal pneumonia, medical unit calls 152, 154–5

G

GCS (Glasgow Coma Scale) neurological observations 24
Gillick Competence 37
gravity-assisted positioning/ drainage 258, 260–2
Guillain-Barré syndrome 185–8

H

haematology patient, case study 286–7
head-injured patient 178–83
health and safety issues, on call policy/procedures 7
heart failure and pulmonary oedema, chest X-ray interpretation 64–5
Hickman catheter 212
high dependency unit (HDU) 3
hip fracture 165
history see patient assessment
huffing technique 237, 238, 239–40
humidification 250–1
hypercapnia
acute-on-chronic respiratory/ ventilatory failure 120
and increased work of breathing 105, 106
causes of acute ventilatory failure 116–17
causes of chronic ventilatory failure 119–20
in Type II respiratory failure 111, 115, 116–19
medications for chronic ventilatory failure 120
signs and symptoms of CO_2 retention 116
treatments 117–19
see also carbon dioxide retention
hypoxaemia (Type I respiratory failure)
acute lobar pneumonia 114
aim of physiotherapy 113
and increased work of breathing 106, 107
bronchopneumonia 114
causes 112
classification 112
clinical signs 113
common issues 113, 114–15

definition 111, 112
treatment of hypoxia 113,
    114–15
use of NIV 91
hypoxia
  and increased work of
    breathing 106, 107
  consequence of decreased V_T
    89
  response in children 38, 44
  treatment for 113, 114–15
  see also hypoxaemia
hypoxic hypoxaemia 112

I

IABP (intra-aortic balloon
    pump) 190
ICP (intracranial pressure)
    values 179, 181
incentive spirometer 251–2
induced sputum 267
induction, preparation for on
    call working 8–9
infected fluid in the lung,
    chest X-ray interpretation
    59, 63
infection, SIRS (systemic
    inflammatory response to
    infection) 131
infection control, on call
    policy/procedures 7, 8
inhaled foreign body, children
    48
intensive care unit (ICU) 3 *see
    also* adult intensive care
    unit (ICU); paediatric
    intensive care unit (PICU)
intermittent positive pressure
    breathing *see* IPPB
interstitial lung disease,
    medical unit calls 149,
    153
interstitial pneumonia 152,
    154
interstitial pulmonary oedema,
    chest X-ray interpretation
    66–7
intra-aortic balloon pump
    (IABP) 190
intracranial pressure (ICP)
    values 179, 181
IPPB (intermittent positive
    pressure breathing) 252–4
  contraindication in
    pneumothorax 67
  risks with COPD 69
ischaemic hypoxaemia 112

K

Kerley B lines, chest X-ray
    interpretation 66, 67

L

laryngectomy patient 167–8
Lasting Power of Attorney
    (LPA) 15–16
lateral costal breathing
    (thoracic expansion) 237,
    238, 239
learning contracts 2–3
learning diary/learning log 4–5
learning from on call events
    3–6
  case studies 5
  critical incident report 4, 5
  debrief afterwards 3–4
  demonstration of what has
    been learned 4
  learning diary/learning log
    4–5
  mentoring 5
  peer review 5
  portfolio of evidence 4–5
  recording your thoughts
    afterwards 3
  reflection on action 4
  reflective diary 3
learning needs assessment (for
    on call working) 1, 2, 8
lobar collapse
  adult intensive care patient
    134
  chest X-ray interpretation
    54–7, 59
  management of volume loss
    97
  signs and symptoms of
    volume loss 92
lobar/multilobar pneumonia,
    medical unit calls 152,
    154
lung abnormalities *see* chest X-
    ray interpretation
    (abnormalities)
lung anatomy *see* chest X-ray
    interpretation (normal)
lung collapse
  chest X-ray interpretation 54,
    58–9
  management of volume loss
    96
  signs and symptoms of
    volume loss 92
lung compliance, effects of
    decreased FRC 87–8

lung contusions 200, 201, 202
  chest X-ray interpretation 59,
    60, 61–2
lung pathology, common ICU
    conditions 131–2
lung volume loss 85–100
  and increased work of
    breathing 106, 107
  ARDS/acute lung injury 92,
    96
  assessment 90, 91–4
  atelectasis 92, 97
  chest X-ray interpretation
    54–9, 63
  clinical diagnosis 90, 92–4
  closing volume 85, 87
  collapse 92, 96
  collapse (lobar) 92, 97
  consolidation 92, 96
  effects of positioning 91
  flail chest 93, 98
  forced vital capacity (FVC)
    85, 86, 89–90
  functional residual capacity
    (FRC) 85–9, 95
  management by diagnosis
    90, 96–100
  pain as cause 93, 98
  patient assessment 18, 19, 36
  pleural effusion 93, 99
  pneumonia 96
  pneumothorax 93, 99
  principles of treatment 90,
    95
  pulmonary oedema 94, 99
  respiratory muscle weakness/
    fatigue 94, 99
  signs and symptoms 90,
    92–4
  tidal volume (V_T) 85, 86, 87,
    89, 90, 95
  underlying
    pathophysiological
    mechanisms 90, 91
  use of CPAP 91, 95–100
  use of NIV 91, 95–100
lung volumes
  closing volume 85, 87
  expiratory reserve volume
    (ERV) 85, 86
  forced vital capacity (FVC)
    85, 86, 89–90
  functional residual capacity
    (FRC) 85–9, 95
  inspiratory capacity (IC) 86
  inspiratory reserve volume
    (IRV) 86

residual volume (RV) 85, 86
tidal volume (V$_T$) 85, 86, 87,
    89, 90, 95
total lung capacity (TLC) 86
vital capacity (VC) 86 *see also*
    forced vital capacity (FVC)

M

manual hyperinflation 242–3
manual insufflation exsufflation
    247
maxillofacial surgery patient 168
mean arterial pressure (MAP)
    values 179
medical staff communication
    with 13
medical unit calls 145–57
    acute asthma 147–8
    bronchiectasis 157
    case study 276–9
    COPD 145–7
    cystic fibrosis (adult) 153,
        155–6
    interstitial lung disease 149,
        153
    oesophageal varices 149, 152
    pancreatitis 149–50
    pneumonia 152, 154–5
    pulmonary fibrosis 149, 153
    renal failure 149, 151–2
Mental Capacity Act (2005)
    (England and Wales)
    15–16
Mental Health Act (1983) 14
mentoring, learning from on
    call events 5
mobilization of patients 254,
    255
MRSA 156
mucociliary clearance, impaired
    73–7
mucolytic drugs 74, 109
musculoskeletal assessment 26
myasthenia gravis 185–6

N

NAI (non-accidental injury) 44,
    48
needlestick injury 8
neonatal unit calls 227–35
    aims of treatment 228
    assessment 232
    common conditions in
        neonates and term babies
        229
    common issues and advice
        230–1

common respiratory
    problems 229
consent 232
decision to treat or not 227
definition of a neonate 227
definition of a premature
    baby 227
definition of a term baby
    227
normal values for neonatal
    vital signs 228
risk factors in treating these
    infants 227–8, 233
techniques contraindicated in
    neonates 234
treatment contraindications
    232
treatment precautions 232
treatment risks to be
    considered 227–8, 233
treatment techniques and
    modifications 233–4
what to ask at the call out
    231
neurological observations,
    patient assessment 24–5
neurological/neurosurgical unit
    calls 177–88
    airway protection 177–8
    brain-injured patient 178–83
    case study 282–4
    causes of respiratory failure
        177
    cerebral perfusion pressure
        (CPP) values 179, 181
    features of a patent airway
        177
    features of inadequate
        ventilation 178
    Guillain-Barré syndrome
        185–8
    head-injured patient 178–83
    intracranial pressure (ICP)
        values 179, 181
    mean arterial pressure (MAP)
        values 179
    myasthenia gravis 185–6
    neurological conditions
        178–88
    neuromedical patient 185–8
    neuromuscular disorders
        178, 185–8
    peripheral neuropathies 178,
        185–8
    respiratory management of
        the neurological patient
        177–8

spinal-injured patient 178,
    183–5
neuromedical patient 185–8
neuromuscular disorders 178,
    185–8
neurophysiological facilitation
    of respiration 254
NIV (non-invasive ventilation)
    255–7
    contraindication in
        pneumothorax 67
    risks with COPD 69
    use in lung volume loss 91,
        95–100
nursing staff, communication
    with 13

O

oesophageal varices 115, 149,
    152
on call competency check list
    2
on call event
    capacity issues 14–16
    communication issues 13–14
    communication with the
        medical/nursing staff 13
    communication with the
        patient/relatives 13
    consent issues 14–16
    disagreement among
        clinicians 13–14
    documentation 16
    patients without capacity (to
        make decisions) 14–16
    things to consider and
        prepare 13–16
    when to seek help 14
    see also learning from on call
        events; preparation for an
        on call event
on call period, on call policy/
    procedures 7
on call policy/procedures 7–8
on call rota
    appropriate and
        inappropriate calls 10, 12
    arrangements on the day of
        your on call 10
    management of the
        telephone call 10–12
    on call logistics 10
    preparation for 9–12
on call working, quality
    standards 1
oncology unit calls 205–14
    anaemia 208

anxiety of patients and relatives 205
ascites 212
aspergillosis 209
assessing patients with an oncology diagnosis 205–6
bony metastatic disease 210–11
cancer treatment modalities 205
case study 288–9
causes of respiratory compromise 205–6
disseminated intravascular coagulation (DIC) 210
effects of acute oncology 208–10
effects of bone marrow depression 207–8
effects of metastatic oncology 210–12
equipment used in the cancer setting 212
Hickman catheter 212
hypercalcaemia 211
lymphangitis carcinomatosa 212
mucositis 208–9
neutropenia 207
PICC line 212
pleural effusion 211
Pneumocystis carinii pneumonia (PCP) 209
pneumonitis 209
side effects of chemotherapy 207–8
spinal cord compression 210
superior vena cava obstruction (SVCO) 211
syringe driver 212
terminal phase of care 212–13
thrombocytopenia 207
tumour occluding airway 208
orthopaedic surgery patient 165–6
orthopaedic trauma 132
osteoporosis 165
overpressure technique 257
oxygen delivery devices for children 47
oxygen demand in infants 38
oxygen therapy 257–8

P
paediatric care
    airway differences 40, 41
anatomical and physiological differences to adults 37–49
assessing children 44–7
auscultation 44, 47
basal metabolic rate in infants 38
bradycardia response to hypoxia 38
child protection 37, 44, 48
chronic respiratory problems 41
clinical implications of anatomical and physiological differences 38–42
common conditions 44, 48
communicating with a child 38
communicating with parents 38
consent issues 37
cyanosis 44
dealing with children 16
hypoxia response 38, 44
information from medical history 43
NAI (non-accidental injury) 44, 48
objective information 44, 46
oxygen delivery devices 47
oxygen demand in infants 38
parents' reactions 38
refusal of treatment 37
signs of respiratory distress 41–2, 44, 49
stridor 41
subjective information 43, 44, 45
sudden infant death syndrome risk 41
thoracic differences 38–9, 41
paediatric intensive care unit (PICU) calls 137–44
    age range of patients 137
aims of physiotherapy 138
airways 139
case study 274–5
common issues in treatment 139–40
inappropriate calls 138
inhaled nitric oxide (NO) 139
oxygen 139–40
range of conditions seen on PICU 137, 142–3
supporting parents 137
treatment precautions 141
ventilation 139–40
paediatric medical ward calls see paediatric unit calls
paediatric surgical ward calls see paediatric unit calls
paediatric unit calls 215–26
    aims of physiotherapy treatment 218
assessment 215, 217–18
assessment (medical ward) 221, 223
assessment (surgical ward) 221–2
case study 289–91
common conditions (medical ward) 222, 225–6
common conditions (surgical ward) 221–2
common issues and advice (medical ward) 222, 224
common issues and advice (surgical ward) 220–1
common problems (medical ward) 223
common problems (surgical ward) 219
conditions requiring extreme caution 215, 216
consent in paediatrics 215
contraindications for treatment 215, 216
inappropriate calls 215, 216
monitors and equipment (surgical ward) 222
paediatric medical ward calls 222–6
paediatric surgical ward calls 218–22
see also paediatric intensive care unit (PICU) calls
pain, as cause of lung volume loss 93, 98
pain management 77, 80
palpation 30
pancreatitis, medical unit calls 149–50
pandemic pneumonia 155
parents
    communicating with 38
    reactions of 38
patient
    communication with 13
    things to consider when called 13–16

unable to cooperate 77, 81
patient assessment 17–36
  ABC assessment 17–18
  auscultation 32–4
  cardiovascular observations 22–3
  changes during assessment 34
  chest pain 20
  chest X-ray interpretation 28–30
  considered approach to assessment 21
  cough 20
  decision-making process 17–18, 19
  drug history 20–1
  early warning scores 34–5
  ECG monitoring 23–4
  four key respiratory problems to look for 18, 19
  general observations 21–2
  history of present condition 18, 20
  immediate danger to the patient 17–18, 19
  increased work of breathing 18, 19, 36
  loss of lung volume 18, 19, 36
  musculoskeletal assessment 26
  neurological observations 24–5
  objective history 21
  palpation 30
  past medical history 20
  percussion note 32
  potential problem list 36
  renal observations 24, 25
  respiratory failure 18, 19, 36
  respiratory observations 26–34
  shortness of breath 20
  social history 21
  sputum 20
  sputum retention 18, 19, 36
  subjective history 18
  surface anatomy/surface marking 30–1
  wheeze 20
peer review, learning from on call events 5
PEP (positive expiratory pressure) mask 240–1
percussion note 32
percussion technique 258

peripheral neuropathies 178, 185–8
peripheral vascular disease 165
personal development plan (PDP) 2
personal risk assessment 8
pharyngeal suction 269–70
PICC line 212
plastic surgery patient 166
pleural effusion
  adult intensive care patient 134
  chest X-ray interpretation 63–4, 65, 66
  lung volume loss 93, 99
Pneumocystis carinii pneumonia (PCP) 154, 209
Pneumocystis jerovici infection 154–5
pneumonectomy, chest X-ray interpretation 54, 58
pneumonia
  bronchopneumonia 152, 154
  chest X-ray interpretation 59, 63
  children 48
  fungal 152, 154–5
  ICU conditions 131–2
  interstitial 152, 154
  lobar/multilobar 152, 154
  lung volume loss 96
  medical unit calls 152, 154–5
  pandemic 155
  PCP (Pneumocystis carinii pneumonia) 154, 209
  Pneumocystis jerovici infection 154–5
  SARS 155
pneumothorax
  adult intensive care patient 134
  chest X-ray interpretation 66–8, 69
  contraindication for positive pressure ventilation 67
  lung volume loss 93, 99
portfolio, evidence of learning from on call events 4–5
positioning
  gravity-assisted drainage 258, 260–2
  positions of ease 258–60
  postural drainage 258, 260–2
  prone 264–5
  to increase volume 263
  to match ventilation/ perfusion ratio 263–4

positions of ease 258–60
positive expiratory pressure (PEP) mask 240–1
positive pressure ventilation
  contraindication in pneumothorax 67
  risks with COPD 69
postoperative patients, ICU calls 133
postoperative respiratory dysfunction, increased WOB 106, 108
postural drainage 258, 260–2
power of attorney 15–16
preparation for an on call event 2–3
  arrange for an induction 3
  learning contracts 2–3
  learning needs assessment 2
  on call competency check list 2
  reflection 2
  spend time on the ICU and HDU 3
  SWOT analysis 2
preparation for on call working 7–9
  clinical experience 8–9
  contractual issues 8
  health and safety issues 7
  identification of learning needs 8
  infection control 7, 8
  on call period 7
  on call policy/procedures 7–8
  on call rota 9–12
  personal risk assessment 8
  referral criteria 7
  response time 7
  shadow duties 9
  things to consider when called to a patient 13–16
  training/induction 8–9
professional bodies, standards for on call working 1
prone positioning 264–5
protective equipment 8
Pseudomonas aeruginosa 156
pulmonary embolus
  adult intensive care patient 134
  hypoxaemia 115
pulmonary fibrosis
  hypoxaemia 115
  medical unit calls 149, 153

pulmonary oedema
    adult intensive care patient
        134
    chest X-ray interpretation 59,
        61, 64–6, 67
    hypoxaemia 115
    increased work of breathing
        108
    lung volume loss 94, 99
Pulmozyme 74

R

recovery room/theatre calls
    168–9
referral criteria, on call policy/
    procedures 7
reflection, preparation for an
    on call event 2
reflection on action 4
reflective diary 3
relatives, communication with
    13
relaxation techniques 266
relaxed tidal breathing 237–8,
    239
renal failure
    hypoxaemia 115
    ICU calls 133
    medical unit calls 149,
        151–2
renal observations, patient
    assessment 24, 25
replacement joint dislocation
    risk 166
respiratory acidosis,
    consequence of decreased
    V_T 89
respiratory assessment see
    patient assessment
respiratory distress, signs in
    children 41–2, 44, 49
respiratory failure
    acute 111
    arterial blood gas tensions
        111
    consequences of 111
    definitions 111
    hypoxaemia (Type I
        respiratory failure) 91,
        106, 107, 111–13, 114–15
    management 111–21
    patient assessment 18, 19, 36
    types of 111, 112
    ventilatory failure (Type II
        respiratory failure) 91,
        105, 106, 111, 113,
        116–20

respiratory failure, Type I
    (hypoxaemia) 111–13,
        114–15
    and increased work of
        breathing 106, 107
    use of NIV 91
respiratory failure, Type II
    (ventilatory failure) 91,
        111, 113, 116–20
    acute-on-chronic respiratory/
        ventilatory failure 120
    causes of acute ventilatory
        failure 116–17
    causes of chronic ventilatory
        failure 119–20
    hypercapnia 111, 113,
        116–20
    increased work of breathing
        105, 106
    medications for chronic
        ventilatory failure 120
    signs and symptoms of CO_2
        retention 113, 116
    treatment of hypercapnia
        117–19
respiratory medical patients,
    ICU calls 133
respiratory muscle efficiency,
    and work of breathing 101
respiratory
    muscle weakness/fatigue
    increased work of breathing
        105
    lung volume loss 94, 99
respiratory muscles, effects of
    decreased FRC 87–8
respiratory physiotherapy
    treatments 237–70
    abdominal breathing 237,
        238, 239
    Acapella device 240–1
    active cycle of breathing
        techniques (ACBT) 237–40
    adjuncts 240–1
    assisted cough 245–7
    autogenic drainage 241
    bagging technique 242–3
    breathing control 237–8, 239
    continuous positive airway
        pressure (CPAP) 248–9
    Cornet (R.C. Cornet®) device
        240–1
    cough 244
    cough, assisted 245–7
    cough assist device 247
    cough stimulation/tracheal
        rub 248

deep breathing exercises 237,
    238, 239
diaphragmatic breathing
    237–8, 239
endotracheal suction 267–9
Flutter device 240–1
forced expiration technique
    (FET) 237, 238, 239–40
gravity-assisted positioning/
    drainage 258, 260–2
huffing 237, 238, 239–40
humidification 250–1
importance of training 237
incentive spirometer 251–2
induced sputum 267
intermittent positive pressure
    breathing (IPPB) 252–4
lateral costal breathing
    (thoracic expansion) 237,
        238, 239
manual hyperinflation
    242–3
manual insufflation
    exsufflation 247
mobilization 254, 255
neurophysiological
    facilitation of respiration
    254
non-invasive ventilation
    (NIV) 255–7
overpressure 257
oxygen therapy 257–8
PEP (positive expiratory
    pressure) mask 240–1
percussion 258
pharyngeal suction 269–70
positioning 258–65
positioning for gravity-
    assisted drainage 258,
        260–2
positioning for postural
    drainage 258, 260–2
positioning to increase
    volume 262–3
positioning to match
    ventilation/perfusion ratio
    263
positions of ease 258–60
positive expiratory pressure
    (PEP) mask 240–1
postural drainage 258, 260–2
prone positioning 264–5
relaxation techniques 266
relaxed tidal breathing
    237–8, 239
rib springing 266–7
saline nebulizer 250–1

shaking technique 267
sputum induction 267
suction, endotracheal 267–9
suction, pharyngeal 269–70
thoracic expansion exercises 237, 238, 239
tracheal rub (cough stimulation) 248
vibrations 270
response time, on call policy/ procedures 7
rib fractures 198, 201, 202
rib springing technique 266–7
risk assessment, personal protection 8
round pneumonia, chest X-ray interpretation 63

S

saline nebulizer 250–1
SARS (severe acute respiratory syndrome) 155
secretions, excessive, sputum retention management 73–7
sepsis 131
complication of pancreatitis 150
shadow duties, preparation for on call working 9
shaking technique 267
SIRS (systemic inflammatory response to infection) 131, 150
spinal injuries 132, 178, 183–5
splash incident to eyes or mouth 8
sputum induction 267
sputum retention
adult intensive care patient 134
clinical signs 71–2
increased work of breathing 109
patient assessment 18, 19, 36
potential causes 71, 73
sputum retention management 71–84
bronchospasm 83
dehydration 77, 82
excessive secretions/impaired mucociliary clearance 73–7
fatigued patient with increased work of breathing 76–7
ineffective cough 77, 78–9
pain management 77, 80

patient unable to cooperate 77, 81
stab injuries 200, 201, 202
standards for on call working 1
stridor, in children 41
suction
endotracheal 267–9
pharyngeal 269–70
sudden infant death syndrome risk 41
surface anatomy/surface marking, patient assessment 30–1
surgical unit, case study 279–82
surgical ward calls 159–75
advising staff on basic management 164
aortic aneurysm 165
arterial bypass graft 165
assessment of the surgical patient 159–62
axillo-femoral bypass 165
ENT surgery patient 167
external fixators 166
facial/intra-oral reconstruction 168
femoro-popliteal bypass 165
general surgery patient 162–4
general surgery treatment precautions 164
hip fracture 165
laryngectomy patient 167–8
major abdominal surgery patient 162–4
maxillofacial surgery patient 168
orthopaedic surgery patient 165–6
osteoporosis 165
peripheral vascular disease 165
plastic surgery patient 166
recovery room calls 168–9
replacement joint dislocation risk 166
rib/sternal injuries 198, 201, 202
spinal injuries 132, 178, 183–5
theatre/recovery room calls 168–9
vascular surgery patient 165
ward-based tracheostomy patient 169–75 *see also* laryngectomy

SWOT analysis, preparation for an on call event 2
syringe driver 212

T

telephone calls
appropriate and inappropriate calls 10, 12
documentation 12
management of 10–12
questions to ask 10, 11 *see also specific conditions*
tension pneumothorax, chest X-ray interpretation 66–8
theatre/recovery room calls 168–9
thoracic cage, effects of disrupted integrity 105
thoracic differences in children 38–9, 41
thoracic expansion exercises 237, 238, 239
thoracic surgery patient 191, 196–98, 199, 200–1
thoracic unit, case study 285–6
thoracotomy, chest X-ray interpretation 54
tidal volume (V_T) 85, 86, 87, 89, 90, 95
causes of decreased V_T 89
consequences of decreased V_T 89
toxic hypoxaemia 112
tracheal rub (cough stimulation) 248
tracheostomy patient (ward-based) 169–75
blocked tracheostomy tube (emergency) 174
common tracheostomy problems 173–4
displaced tracheostomy tube (emergency) 174–5
emergency situations 174–5
essential equipment 170–1
haemorrhage (emergency) 173, 174, 175
indications for tracheostomy 170
local protocols for tracheostomy care 169
methods of tracheostomy tube insertion 169
mini-tracheostomy 169, 170, 171, 172
percutaneous tracheostomy 169

surgical tracheostomy 169
types of tracheostomy tube
170, 171, 172
see also laryngectomy
training in respiratory
physiotherapy treatments
237
training/induction, preparation
for on call working 8–9
traumatic lung contusion, chest
X-ray interpretation 59, 60,
61–2
treatment options *see*
respiratory physiotherapy
treatments
Type I respiratory failure *see*
respiratory failure, Type I
(hypoxaemia)
Type II respiratory failure *see*
respiratory failure, Type II
(ventilatory failure)

V

V_T (tidal volume) 85, 86, 87,
89, 90, 95

vaccination record (personal
protection) 8
vascular surgery patient 165
ventilation/perfusion ratio,
positioning to match 263
ventilatory failure *see*
respiratory failure, Type II
vibrations (respiratory
physiotherapy treatment)
270
volume, positioning to increase
262–3
volume loss *see* lung volume
loss
volumes *see* lung volumes

W

whooping cough (pertussis),
children 48
work of breathing (WOB)
definition 101
during quiet respiration
101
effects of reduced respiratory
muscle efficiency 101

work of breathing (WOB),
increased 101–9
bronchospasm treatments
101, 103–4
clinical signs 101, 102–3
disrupted integrity of the
thoracic cage 105
hypercapnia and Type II
respiratory failure 105, 106
hypoxia and Type I
respiratory failure 106, 107
oral mucolytics 109
patient assessment 18, 19, 36
reduced respiratory muscle
efficiency 101
respiratory muscle weakness
105
sputum retention
management 76–7
volume loss (static and
dynamic) 106, 107

X

X-rays *see* chest X-ray
interpretation